AN ABC OF PROSTATE CANCER IN 2015

My Journey over 4 Continents

to Find the Best Cure

Alan G. Lawrenson

First Edition – Copyright © 2014 Alan G. Lawrenson

Published by Alan G. Lawrenson, Pretty Beach, NSW, Australia

Design and Layout by Alan G. Lawrenson

ISBN: 978-1507671771

Printed by CreateSpace, An Amazon.com Company

Disclaimer: Every care has been taken in preparing this book to present information fully, accurately and correctly. The author takes **NO RESPONSIBILITY** for any information that might not be accurate and correct, fully covered or excluded, either intentionally or in error. Furthermore, the information in this book is provided under the understanding that the author is not rendering medical advice. The sole purpose of this book is to assist the reader to ask informed questions of their qualified healthcare professionals. **IT IS IMPERATIVE THAT ALL PERSONS READING THIS BOOK, SHOULD SEEK THE SERVICES OF EXPERIENCED AND APPROPRIATE MEDICAL PROFESSIONALS TO DIAGNOSE AND/OR TREAT ANY CONDITION, DISEASE OR MALADY THAT THEY MAY OR MAY NOT HAVE.** The author of this book is not a medical doctor, and the reader is advised that any information or opinions expressed or implied in this book are those of a layman and should not be acted upon without the consent of a qualified medical professional. The author is expressly not liable for any damages or negative consequences that might follow from any treatment, actions or procedures undertaken by any person or persons reading or following the contents, information or opinions within this book, including the research papers referred to in the book.

All rights reserved. No part of this publication may be reproduced, stored in a retrieval system, or transmitted in any form or by any means, electronic, mechanical, photocopying, recording, or otherwise, without the prior written permission of the publisher.

DEDICATION

This book is dedicated to two people:

Dudley C. R. Clear

He was my English master from 1958 to 1962 at the Grey High School in Port Elizabeth, South Africa. He instilled in me a great liking of the English language; how it ought to be written and spoken. His English skills rubbed off on me to a substantial extent. This has allowed me to progress through life with a good command of the spoken and written word. He was more than a teacher: he was a Master of his craft. His tutoring and guidance instilled in me the desire to be an author one day. It has taken 52 years to achieve this goal.

Douglas J. Simmons

Doug, as he was affectionately known, became a work colleague in 1980. He was the second person that I had known who succumbed to prostate cancer. He was one of the bravest men I have known. I was with him the day he returned from the specialist and informed us that he was expected to die from the disease within two years. He fought the cancer battle with courage, strength and dignity, displaying a determination to continue his contribution to the company within the confines of his health.

After I was diagnosed with prostate cancer in 2012, I reflected again on the extent of the illness that claimed his life in 1983 at the all-too-young age of 55. It belatedly provided added encouragement for me to write this book.

If the contents of this book can help spare only one person from going through what Doug bravely endured, then my efforts would be well worth it.

A FINAL MESSAGE

ALL MEN FROM THE AGE OF 40 SHOULD UNDERGO REGULAR PSA AND DRE TESTING

CONTENTS

Dedication 3

What this book is and what it is not 6

PART 1: MY INITIAL DIAGNOSIS

Chapter 1.   I am diagnosed with Prostate Cancer 10

Chapter 2.   What is Prostate Cancer................................. 16

Chapter 3.   How is Prostate Cancer detected?................. 22

PART 2: TREATMENT OPTIONS

Chapter 4.   Introductory Comments on Treatment Options 47

Chapter 5.   Active Surveillance or Watchful Waiting 51

Chapter 6.   Surgery 55

Chapter 7.   Radiation 64

    7.1   External Beam Radiation Therapy (EBRT) 64

    7.2   3-D CRT, IMRT, IGRT and Tomography 69

    7.3   Stereotactic Body Radiotherapy (SBRT)............... 74

    7.4   Proton Beam Therapy 79

    7.5   Low Dose Brachytherapy (Seeds)......................... 94

    7.6   High Dose Brachytherapy................................... 102

Chapter 8.   Hyperthermia 109

Chapter 9.   Cryosurgery 117

Chapter 10. High Intensity Focussed Ultrasound (HIFU) 123

Chapter 11. Focal Laser Ablation 130

Chapter 12. Hormone Therapy 136

Chapter 13. Chemotherapy and Immunotherapy 146

Chapter 14. Complementary and Alternative Therapies.............. 153

Chapter 15. The Role of Support Groups 172

PART 3: MY PROSTATE CANCER EXPERIENCE

Chapter 16.	My Prostate Cancer: Ongoing Research	177
Chapter 17.	Was HIFU the Answer?	182
Chapter 18.	A Third Urologist Enters the Picture	184
Chapter 19.	Proton Beam Therapy Re-Visited	188
Chapter 20.	Enter the Radiation Oncologist	190
Chapter 21.	Enter the Case for Hyperthermia	192
Chapter 22.	How Do You Get to a Final Treatment Decision?	198
Chapter 23.	The Decision: Proton Beam Therapy in Korea	201
Chapter 24.	The Pre-Treatment Program in Korea	204
Chapter 25.	My Treatment Begins	211
Chapter 26.	The Post Treatment Period	214
Chapter 27.	Would I Make the Same Decision Again?	216
Appendix 1.	Glossary	221
Appendix 2.	Abbreviations	247
Appendix 3.	Resource Listings	249
Appendix 4.	Reference Listings	253
Appendix 5.	Proton Beam Therapy Centres	268
Appendix 6.	Acknowledgements	285

INTRODUCTION

What this Book is and What it is Not

This book is about a number of things.

Firstly, it tells the story of me being diagnosed with intermediate stage prostate cancer. This level of prostate cancer needs active medical intervention. Unnecessary delays could result in the cancer developing into the advanced localised stage or worse, over time, into life threatening metastatic prostate cancer.

Secondly, it examines the ten treatment options that are available to prostate cancer sufferers today, plus subsets of some of these treatments, e.g. there are 9 forms of radiation therapy discussed in this book. It includes details of the most common treatments and others that are a little less so. With the possible exclusion of complementary and alternative medicine, all these treatments are being practised daily by medical professionals around the world. All have been subjected to significant research and scrutiny and almost all have been the subject of successful randomised clinical trials.

All information in this book has been based on my own experiences or from my **very extensive search of the information on prostate cancer that is in the public domain.** This has included books on prostate cancer, web sites of hospitals, universities and research institutes, government bodies such as the US National Institute of Health, not-for-profit bodies such as the Australian Cancer Council, proceedings from learned societies, other web sites, blog sites, testimony by fellow prostate cancer suffers, input from medical practitioners (both physicians and surgeons) and other reliable sources.

Thirdly, it outlines the process I went through, to find the best treatment option to suit my particular circumstances. It also details the actual treatment process that I underwent. Finally, I look back at my treatment and whether I would make the same selection again after reviewing the outcomes achieved and the new information gleaned in the process of researching and writing this book.

Hopefully you will find this book an interesting and informative read. I also hope that it will give prostate cancer sufferers and their families, a wider general overview of the processes and procedures that might be available to them and prepare them, more fully, to effectively engage with their medical team.

What this book is NOT, is medical advice. I am NOT a doctor, nor have I been trained in medicine. Thus, it is imperative that all prostate cancer sufferers, their families and supporters, who read this book, seek appropriate medical advice from medical professionals.

Every patient has differing characteristics and circumstances that can only be assessed by competent medical professionals. Reading this book may be helpful in at least providing useful background information that might assist in the critically important patient/doctor dialogue, which is so necessary at every stage of the journey to beat the cancer. The questions listed in the book under various treatment options might be appropriate for some patients, but not for others. Take from the book what you will, but beyond all else, take heed of what your medical team are recommending and act on it appropriately.

All care has been taken in preparing this book to present information fully, accurately and correctly. I take NO RESPONSIBILITY for any information that might not be accurate and correct, fully covered or excluded, either intentionally or in error.

Things are moving very quickly in the prostate cancer treatment field. What was good advice yesterday, might not be so tomorrow. New information comes available every day! I have had difficulty in deciding what new or relatively new information to include. Tomorrow might see the announcement of a significant breakthrough. Thus I have drawn a line under what is to be included in this text. Hopefully, this book will be a success and I will be encouraged to update its content within a few years.

What background or training equipped me to write what is partially a technical review of treatments that are available for prostate cancer?

After being tertiary educated in the physical sciences, I worked in the commercial side of science for 46 years before retiring in 2006. Much of the last decade until 2006, was spent as the chief executive of an organisation called Science Industry Australia Inc. The SIA, as it was often referred to, was (and still is) a peak industry body, whose core purpose was/is the growth of the science industry in Australia. I was extensively involved with the Australia Federal Government in the establishment and implementation of the Science Industry Action Agenda and the Medical Devices Action Agenda. These Action Agendas were the mechanism used by the then John Howard's Coalition Government, to grow the commercialisation output of scientific and medical research institutes, universities and hospitals into products or services that could be marketed by these two industries, locally and internationally. I also spent 10 years attending the Board of the peak umbrella body of scientific and medical research professional societies from 1995 to 2006. Over a 25 year period, I had the privilege to attend more than 100 scientific and medical conferences in Australia, the USA, the UK, Japan, Singapore, Germany and South Africa. These activities have seen me develop an ability to translate technical research findings into more simplified documents that could be understood by non-scientific or non-medical personnel.

The book was written for three main reasons. Firstly, I aimed to provide what I believe to be a comprehensive review of the "state of play" in the treatment of prostate cancer. Secondly, I hope to perhaps assist newly-diagnosed patients to pause and to take a step back, whilst they are in what I call "Cancer Anxiety Factor" mode. It is very difficult to consider the treatment options offered them by their medical specialists or other alternatives, when faced with the psychological pressure to immediately rid oneself of the cancer. One needs time to weigh up the advantages and disadvantages of the various options available. Thirdly, I feel that proton beam therapy (and some of the lesser known treatment options) presents men with perhaps greater certainty of outcome compared to surgery, x-ray radiation or brachytherapy.

The sub-title of the book is *"My Journey over 4 Continents to find the Best Cure"*. Many doctors will tell you that there is no such thing as a "cure" for cancer, but there is only "remission" from the cancer. I don't disagree with this point of view, but find it easier to use the word "cure" in the title. Finally, after much consideration, I decided not to identify any of the doctors in this book by name, other than Dr Cho Kwan-Ho, who was responsible for my treatment at the National Cancer Centre's proton beam facility in Korea. I can say that all the doctors that I came across in my journey, were highly competent and had my best interests at heart. My use of an initial to identify them, should not suggest anything to the reader or indeed the doctor in question (should they read this book)!

One last technical note. Most of the images in this book were sourced as full colour images that might not be as clear when presented in black and white as they are in this book. The colour images will be viewable in colour on the book's web site at www.anabcofprostatecancer.com.au from late February 2015.

PART 1: MY INITIAL DIAGNOSIS

Chapter 1.

I am Diagnosed with Prostate Cancer

It was mid-April 2012. A few days following my biopsy to determine whether or not the acceleration of my PSA (**Prostate Specific Antigen**) reading was due to prostate cancer, I walked into Dr P's rooms to discuss the biopsy results without any real foreboding. After all, my wife, and I were about to jet out of Sydney (Australia) for a four week holiday in South Africa. We had emigrated from there in 1979.

As my late father had prostate cancer for the last 25 years of his life and my brother also has had prostate cancer for the last 12 years, I was a little preconditioned to receiving bad news. Researchers in the 70's had established a significant hereditary link between male family members. In my case, the chances of getting prostate cancer were suggested to me as being as high as 80%. However, an authoritative study suggests the likelihood is actually about 30%.[1]

Dr P, whom I knew as a fellow golfer, said as we sat down *"Alan, you have prostate cancer. The pathologist found that 9 of the 24 rods taken during the biopsy, were cancerous to a lesser or greater extent."* I felt a little stunned to say the least. Where was this news likely to take me?

The rest of the fifteen minute consultation became a bit of a blur. The doctor explained that I had Type 1c prostate cancer with a Gleason score of 3 + 4 = 7. This is an intermediate grade cancer that was likely to grow more rapidly than one with a lower Gleason score of 6 or below, but slower than one with a score of 8 to 10, which are the most aggressive grades. Type 1 and Type 2 prostate cancers are considered to be still confined to the "box" and are likely not to have spread to the seminal glands or other parts of the body.

Dr P then went on to discuss treatment options. These included a prostatectomy or radiation therapy. Of course, not much sank in, as I was in a state of mild shock. He gave me a copy of the Australian Cancer Council's comprehensive 128 page book on prostate cancer titled **"Localised Prostate Cancer – A guide for men and their families"**. (Unfortunately, this book is no longer available in hard or online copy).

I walked out of the doctor's rooms after making an appointment to see him in mid-June 2012 after our return from South Africa. (We returned from South Africa a day or two after Dr P went overseas for a month, thus delaying the next appointment). This delay in considering the next step in choosing my treatment became very important to me, as it gave me time to thoroughly investigate the options available to me.

Of course, the first step was to discuss the matter thoroughly with my wife, Pamela, who had spent almost her whole working life employed as a scrub nurse or as an operating room manager. Not very participatory are wives who are retired nurses!

She did concur with me that I should spend as much time as possible thoroughly researching each realistic available treatment option. The guide referred to above was an excellent starting point. It covers the whole gambit of Localised Prostate Cancer including an array of questions that need to be asked of the medical professional.

My brother, who had been diagnosed with prostate cancer some 12 years earlier, was my first port of call. I had a basic understanding of his treatment, but it was time to find out more specific information. His PSA was then similar to mine at 8.0 and tests showed no signs of the cancer having migrated external of the prostate. He had had exposure to Chinese medicine prior to his cancer diagnosis, and decided to undertake an ongoing course of herbal treatment prescribed by his specialist (who offered conventional treatment as well as Chinese herbal solutions). After 18 months of herbal treatment, his PSA was still elevated, but was not increasing. I am not sure what the catalyst was, but he decided to see Dr S, one of Sydney's leading prostate cancer specialists.

He recommended that my brother undergo high dose rate brachytherapy via the temporary insertion of radioactive-tipped needles into the prostate. This was to be followed by a 6 week course of x-ray radiation. This treatment regime was concluded in early 2003, after which his PSA level dropped over some months, to below 2 ng/ml. This level is generally regarded as men being clear of prostate cancer. He continued to have twice yearly PSA tests done, which were all below 2 until October 2008, when his PSA was up to 3.5, then by October 2009 to 9.28. Clearly, some cancer cells had survived the high dose rate brachytherapy and the follow up x-ray radiation.

His urologist advised that he was not a candidate for further radiation treatment as his urethra (the tube from the bladder to the penis) had become too brittle due to its radiation exposure. He was put on a course of Zoladex®, which is a hormonal therapy, called androgen deprivation therapy or ADT. Over three months this reduced his PSA to 0.51.

ADT causes an increase in the oestrogen to androgen ratio in the body lowering the testosterone and can be accompanied by side effects such as hot flushes, lack of libido and erectile strength, breast swelling and in some cases, nausea. It is usually only taken continually for six months with a similar length break, before one can resume treatment for a further three or six month period. Continuous usage is suggested to reduce its ongoing effectiveness.

From 2011 to 2012, his PSA again increased from 0.78 to 7.94. He began another round of ADT (Zoladex®) and again reverted to Chinese herbal treatment. He also added a course of acupuncture to his treatment program. The herbal treatment was designed to strengthen his T-cells which are the immune system's 'cancer fighters'. This treatment program cost him about US$9,500 (A$10,000) a year. His PSA remained under 1.0 until September 2013, when it nudged up to 1.43. By June 2014, it had risen to 4.55 ng/ml, which started to set off alarm bells. At the time this book goes to press, he has sought a second opinion from a urologist who has an integrated practice which includes their own multiparametric MRI machine (3T) and all the latest whistles and bells. Hopefully, the cancer has not metastasised beyond the immediate prostate region. The possibility of me wanting to undergo brachytherapy with needles, dropped down the list of possible treatments, even though this point of view was based on a sample of only one.

A close friend, John, now 79, had eleven years previously been one of the first Australians to undergo **Proton Beam Therapy** (PBT) at the Loma Linda University Medical Centre in California, USA. This form of radiation therapy uses protons to irradiate the prostate rather than photons that are used in all forms of x-ray radiation. The proton beam is created from hydrogen atoms in a cyclotron that accelerates the protons to about 100,000 miles per hour (160,000 kilometres per hour). The proton beam line, as it is called, is focussed via each hip joint to the prostate. It is considered to be the least damaging of all radiation techniques to the tissue that surrounds the prostate such as the bladder, rectum, seminal glands, etc. John returned from Loma Linda with absolutely minimal peripheral damage and a PSA that quickly dropped below 2. Subsequently, he became the product advocate for a Sydney based company, who hope to build the first PBT facility in Australia. Only 40 such facilities exist internationally at this time, with only one in the Southern Hemisphere in Cape Town, South Africa (which only treats eye and brain cancers).

The drawback of Proton Beam Therapy to Australians, and others distant from a facility that accepts foreign patients, is the cost of the treatment, accommodation and travel and the minimum of 7 weeks (usually 10 weeks) duration of the treatment. Costs range from US$55,000 to more than US$100,000.

I continued to search the internet for information on all the realistic alternatives available to me. There is a massive array of information available and it became a serious task to decipher fact from fiction. I should explain that my disposition causes me a need to obtain as complete a picture of things as possible. Working in science for 46 years sharpened my determination to gather all pertinent facts before deciding on a course of action. I found that the medical profession, in general, only want you to know what they think you should know. This has happened to me time and time again and I find these characteristics of (many) doctors frustrating.

My internet search saw my interest in two techniques escalate to the fore. These were Proton Beam Therapy (PBT) and High Intensity Focussed Ultrasound (HIFU). The latter technique has been around since the late 1990's with two machines being available; the Sonoblate® from Focus Surgery Inc., Indiana, USA and the Ablatherm® from EDAP TMS S.A., Lyon, France. The latter is widely used in Europe and has subsidiaries in Italy, Germany, USA, Japan, Korea and Malaysia. The Sonoblate is used more so in Japan, Australia and other countries. A further HIFU machine is made by a Chinese manufacturer with more than 165 hospitals in China using the local machine. The technique involves heating the prostate via an ultrasonic probe placed in the rectum. It is over in a couple of hours and outcomes are generally excellent.

My research was interrupted when Pam and I journeyed to South Africa to visit friends and relatives. It also allowed me to attend the 50th year Reunion of the Class of 1962, at the Grey High School in Port Elizabeth. A great time was had over the four day celebration which culminated in attendance at the Grey 1st XV Rugby team taking on a visiting team from Cape Town. Four of my closer school chums and I sat together to watch the match and I soon discovered that we all had become victims of prostate cancer. Roy had had brachytherapy seeds implanted; 'Michael' had had a prostatectomy; Graham had EBRT; John didn't want to be specific about his treatment; and I still had to decide my treatment option.

Roy could not urinate for six weeks after his treatment and had to self-insert a catheter to do so. 'Michael' was substantially impotent; Graham had unspecified problems and I suspect John also was not firing on all cylinders. This information again reinforced my desire to make the right choice to manage my condition.

Whilst I was in South Africa, I checked with National Accelerator Centre attached to Tygerberg Hospital, near Cape Town, as to whether or not they had started doing prostate cancer treatment with their proton beam system. Unfortunately, they still focus entirely on cancers of the head and brain stem. If I could have been treated there, I would have had free accommodation at one of Pam's relatives, who lives nearby the Centre!

On our mutual returns from our travels, my first urologist and I discussed options. He preferred to do a complete prostatectomy (his speciality!), but I wanted a second opinion from a highly credentialed urologist at a Sydney cancer institute with whom I was familiar. Dr L was also one of only a few practitioners who practice the HIFU procedure.

I now side-track to look at what prostate cancer is, how it is diagnosed and assessed, and to provide information on the latest treatments available. In Chapter 16, I resume my journey to discover the best treatment option available to me.

Chapter 2.
What is Prostate Cancer?

Cancer is a disease in which cells in the body grow out of control. When cancer starts in the prostate, it is called prostate cancer. This malignant cell growth can be localised or advanced. **Localised prostate cancer** refers to those cancers that have not grown beyond the prostate. They generally have few or no symptoms and often do not develop into advanced prostate cancer. **Advanced prostate cancer** generally refers to cancers that have spread beyond the prostate into surrounding tissue and/or into the bones or other parts of the body including lymph nodes. The book referred to in Chapter 1, divides advanced prostate cancer into two groupings: **locally advanced prostate cancer** and advanced prostate cancer. They suggest that locally advanced prostate cancers are those cancers that remain in the immediate region of the prostate (or in the wall of the prostate). Advanced prostate cancers are those that have spread beyond the prostate into the seminal glands and/or the lymph nodes. When advanced prostate cancer spreads to the bones and distant organs it is referred to as **metastatic prostate cancer**.

This book focused substantially on localised and advanced prostate cancer, or as is often stated, prostate cancer that is "still in the box" or in the region immediately adjacent to the prostate. Metastatic prostate cancer is a far more challenging progression of the disease that requires immediate specialist attention. An excellent booklet on metastatic prostate cancer titled *"Living with bone metastases from prostate cancer"* is available for download via Appendix 3.

Apart from skin cancer, prostate cancer is the most common cancer in Australian men. I find the ignorance and/or disinterest displayed by many men in the 60 to 75 year age group about prostate cancer quite remarkable.

It would probably be beneficial to many readers, for us to have a look at what constitutes the prostate. It is a part of the male reproductive system, which includes the penis, the prostate, the seminal glands, and the testicles. The prostate is located just below the bladder and in front of the rectum. It is about the size of a walnut and surrounds the urethra (the tube that empties urine from the bladder). It produces fluid that makes up a part of semen. As a man ages, the prostate tends to increase in size. This can cause the urethra to narrow and decrease urine flow. This is called **benign prostatic hyperplasia** (often referred to as BPH), and it is not the same as prostate cancer. Men may also have other prostate changes that are not cancer.

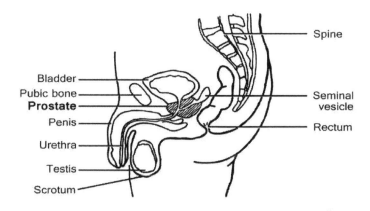

Image: Courtesy of Wikipedia

This diagram shows the location of the prostate, in front of the rectum and just below the bladder. Let's look at the anatomy of the prostate. When looking at the prostate from the front, it can be is divided into four zones. These are:

The outer **peripheral zone (PZ),** which contains between 70% - 80% of the glandular tissue (in young men). The volume of the PZ increases from the base to the apex of the gland.

The **transition zone (TZ)** surrounding the urethra which contains about 5% of the glandular tissue.

The **central zone (CZ)** which has about 20% of the glandular tissue.

The **anterior** (fibro muscular) **zone (AZ)** or stroma, which contains no glandular tissue.

Prostate Zones

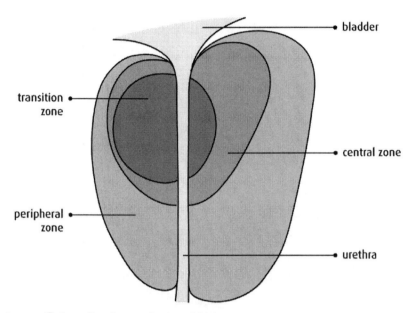

Image: © Canadian Cancer Society 2014

Many medical publications and doctors refer to "lobes" rather than "zones". They correlate broadly as follows:

Anterior lobe (or isthmus) – roughly equates to part of the TZ

Posterior lobe – roughly equates to the PZ

Middle or median lobe – roughly equates to part of the CZ

Lateral lobe – spans all zones.

Prostate cancers usually commence in the glandular tissue of the prostate, with about 70% originating in the PZ, about 25% in the TZ zone, and 5% in the central zone. It is very difficult for imaging to separate, the TZ from the CZ. As a result, these two zones are often referred to together as the central gland.

The prostate does not have a capsule, rather an outer band of fibro muscular tissue that surrounds it. It is integrated with the muscles of the pelvic floor, which contract during the ejaculatory process. The outer layer of tissue in the rear and rear-sides of the gland are more "capsule-like" and are visible as a layer of thin tissue on T2-weighed MRI images. The 'capsule" is important for the assessment of possible **extra-prostatic capsular extension** (ECE) in DRE diagnosis. Hardness, irregularities, bulges, etc. in the capsular tissue suggest a tumour within the prostate or its spread outside the confines of the prostate.

The **neurovascular bundles** "wrap" around the prostate and are seen at the 5-o'clock and 7-o'clock positions in reference to the prostate on imaging. At the top and bottom of the prostate the nerve bundles have branches that penetrate into the capsule. These pathways provide a route for extra-prostatic tumour extension into the neurovascular bundles.

Roughly 20,000 men are diagnosed with prostate cancer each year in Australia with around 3,000 dying from the disease. The good news is that this number is not growing, probably due to increased early detection and post detection medical intervention and treatment. This compares to about 240,000 men being diagnosed each year in the USA. Deaths attributed to prostate cancer in the USA are close to 30,000 per annum with this number likely to increase significantly in coming years due to the active discouraging of PSA testing by governmental panels and medical associations. More information on this shortly.

Age is a significant factor in the incidence of prostate cancer. Only a handful per 1,000 men under the age of 50 are diagnosed with prostate cancer, with the detection rate growing to 24 per 1000 in 50 – 59 year olds; 73 per 1000 in the 60 – 69 age group; increasing to 94 in the 70 – 79 and 93 in the 80 – 89 age groups.[1]

Many men diagnosed with early stage prostate cancer, do not necessarily need active treatment. **Active surveillance** is a commonly recommended way forward.

It is not known what causes prostate cancer to take hold in some men, but not in others. There is a view that diet is a factor in the evolvement of prostate cancer. We explore this further in Chapter 12. There are significant differences in the prevalence of prostate cancer between African-Americans (high prostate cancer) and Japanese (low prostate cancer). Clearly the dietary habits of these two groups are significantly different. About 10% of men who have prostate cancer who have a father and/or brother with early-diagnosed prostate cancer (50 - 59 years old), appear to have a pre-disposition to prostate cancer. This pre-disposition appears to be due to inheriting faulty cancer protection genes, rather than genes themselves causing the cancer. Considerable research is enhancing understanding of the effect of genetics on prostate cancer and the development of other types of cancer. What is clear is that if you have a father with an early prostate cancer diagnosis your chance of developing prostate cancer is doubled and with two near relatives with early prostate cancer diagnosis, your chances of prostate cancer rises seven fold.

Generally, prostate cancer is slow to spread. Of course when it is detected, it might already be well advanced. The following possibilities exist:

The prostate cancer is confined to the prostate only (it's contained "in the box"). This is referred to as localised prostate cancer. Time is on the patient's side, due to generally slow progression of the disease.

It may have spread to other tissue outside the prostate, such as the seminal vesicles. This is often referred to **localised advanced prostate.**

Spread to nearby organs sees it called **advanced prostate cancer.**

Spread to the bones, liver and elsewhere is regarded as **metastatic prostate cancer.**

The last three possibilities listed above, need urgent medical intervention.

From around the age of 50 onwards, most men start to have some difficulties in urinating. They find themselves:

Getting up during the night to pass water (once at first; then twice and eventually more often).

Not being able to "start" to pass water when one needs to go. It's embarrassing to stand at a urinal for up to 5 minutes counting (silently!) from 1 to 100.

Similarly, when the flow stops and starts.

Occasionally, with an over-powering need to urinate immediately.

The cause of much of the above is a non-malignant enlargement of the prostate which is often called benign prostate hyperplasia or BPH. Urologists often treat this condition by surgical intervention by doing a procedure called a **trans-urethral resection (TURP).** I had this "partial rebore" in which the urologist removes material from the urethra area of the prostate to improve urinary flows. More details on this procedure in Chapter 17.

When prostate cancer is an advanced stage, symptoms start to emerge which may include pain during ejaculation; burning when passing water; inability to empty the bladder completely; blood in urine or semen and/or continuing lower back, pelvis or hip pain, or stiffness. A reduction in the quality of holding an erection also occurs in some cases.

Once prostate cancer is diagnosed, most men want to be rid of the disease quickly, by pursuing early treatment. According to the American Cancer Society, the bias toward treatment in the U.S. contrasts sharply with other countries. For example, an estimated 20–30% of European men choose active surveillance compared with only about 5–10% of American men. This early intervention mentality is beyond frustrating to Otis Brawley, MD, chief medical officer of the American Cancer Society, who stated at an AACR conference in early 2014: *"One of the problems I've had with this frenzy of prostate cancer screening and treatment over the last 25 years, is that we've actually impeded scientific development of the new markers we desperately need to figure out the cancers that kill versus the cancers that don't kill."*

Chapter 3.
How is Prostate Cancer Detected?

Testing

Two tests are commonly used to screen for prostate cancer. They are a digital rectal examination (DRE) and a prostate specific antigen (PSA) test. Let's look at them more closely.

Digital rectal exam (DRE):

The prostrate is sited immediately adjacent to the rectum wall. The doctor inserts a gloved, lubricated finger into the rectum to estimate the size of the prostate and feel for lumps or other abnormalities. The DRE can only feel part of the prostate gland and that is the posterior zone adjacent to the rectum. Lumps or other abnormalities present in the anterior region or other prostate areas, which are not reached during the rectal examination, would be missed.

Prostate specific antigen (PSA) test:

This test measures the level of PSA in the blood. The PSA is a protein produced by cells in the prostate. Its primary function is to help keep the semen in a liquid form enabling the sperm to swim. The levels of PSA can rise due to a number of reasons including the presence of cancer. The levels of PSA in the blood can be higher in men who have prostate cancer. The PSA level may also be elevated in other conditions that affect the prostate. The most frequent benign prostate condition that causes an elevation in PSA level is prostatitis - inflammation of the prostate - and benign prostatic hyperplasia (BPH), which we have already read, is the enlargement of the prostate. Some drugs used to treat BPH have been found to lower PSA levels.

As a rule, the higher the PSA level in the blood, the more likely a prostate problem is present. But many factors, such as age and ethnicity, can affect PSA levels. Some prostate glands make more PSA than others. PSA levels also can be affected by:

Certain medical procedures

Certain medications

An enlarged prostate

A prostate infection

Ejaculation within 24 hours of having the test done

Bicycle riding.

Most doctors prescribe a urinary test to check for a possible infection when ordering a PSA test. An infection is likely to elevate the PSA result.

In a large study reported in 2004 by Thompson, et al., it was found that 15% of men who had a prostate that felt normal on examination and a PSA less than 4, went on to be confirmed later in the study by biopsy of having prostate cancer. Of the 15% who had prostate cancer, 33.7% of the 15% had a final PSA of less or equal to 2.0 ng/ml. Participants were aged from 62 to 91 years old.[1] Of course, the higher the age the greater the likelihood of a positive finding. The Boots WebMD web site's Prostate Cancer Guide reports men who have a 'normal' PSA level below 4 ng/ml have a 15% chance of having prostate cancer. Those with a PSA level between four and 10 have a 25% chance of having prostate cancer and if the PSA is higher than 10, the risk increases to 67%.[2,3]

Your doctor is the best person to interpret your PSA test results, because, as we have seen, many factors can affect PSA levels. If the result of the test is abnormal, further testing is needed to see if there is a cancer present. If prostate cancer is suggested as a result of screening with the PSA test or DRE, it will probably be at an earlier, more treatable stage than if no screening were done. If it is decided to do another PSA test a few months down the track, it is important to ensure that the test is done in the same pathology laboratory that did the first test, as there is significant variability in PSA testing between laboratories.

There is no specific normal or abnormal level of PSA in the blood. In the past, most doctors considered PSA levels of 4.0 ng/ml and lower as normal. Therefore, if a man had a PSA level higher than 4.0 ng/ml, doctors would often recommend a prostate biopsy to determine whether or not prostate cancer was present. If there is a family history of prostate cancer and if the PSA level is higher than 2.0 ng/ml, doctors are likely to prescribe regular PSA testing. Neither the PSA test nor the DRE is 100% accurate. These tests can sometimes have abnormal results even when cancer is not present (known as false-positive results). Normal results can also occur even when cancer is present (known as false-negative results). False-positive results often lead to some men having a prostate biopsy (with its attendant risks of pain, infection, and bleeding) when they do not have cancer. False-negative results can give some men a false sense of security even though they actually have cancer.

Another important issue is that even if DRE and/or PSA screening detect cancer, doctors aren't able to ascertain if the cancer is aggressive or passive. Some prostate cancers grow so slowly that they would probably never cause problems or show symptoms of cancer being present. Because of an elevated PSA level, some men may be diagnosed with a prostate cancer that they would have never even known about at all. It would never have led to their death, or even caused any symptoms.

Today, it would be highly unlikely that a doctor would recommend aggressive intervention such as surgery or radiation treatment without the patient undergoing a biopsy. Only after the results of the biopsy are known, can the doctor (urologist) determine the extent of the cancer and it level of "aggressiveness". More details on biopsy testing follow later in this chapter.

Doctors agree that the PSA blood test is not a perfect test for the early detection of prostate cancer. As indicated earlier, a low PSA test value might cause some cancers to be missed, and in other cases it is elevated when cancer isn't present. A PSA result of less than 10 ng/ml, suggests the cancer is likely to be confined to the prostate ("in the box"), with 30 ng/ml or higher readings, suggesting that the cancer might have spread beyond the prostate. Even in cases were the PSA is > 10 ng/ml, the statistics suggest that the likelihood of prostate cancer being present is less than one in three in one study and one in two in another.[4]

Your doctor may order a follow-up PSA test that measures **"free" PSA** (the standard PSA test measures "total" PSA). This test measures the amount of PSA in the blood that is "free" (not bound to other proteins) divided by the total amount of PSA (free plus bound). This is usually expressed as a percentage. Low ratios (less than 15% free to total PSA) suggest a higher risk of cancer being present whilst higher ratios of above 20% free to total PSA, suggest less likelihood of cancer being present. Some evidence suggests that a lower proportion of free PSA may be associated with more aggressive cancer.

Age is a key factor in deciding on future action. DRE and PSA should be undertaken for men over 40 if there has been a family history of prostate cancer. All men over 50 should have a DRE and PSA test undertaken when having their annual physical check-up.

In early 2012, the United States Preventative Services Task Force (USPSTF) came out with an astonishing recommendation: Doctors should abandon routine PSA testing in healthy men. The USPSTF were seriously concerned about the massive over-servicing of prospective and confirmed prostate cancer patients. This included hundreds of thousands of "unnecessary" biopsies, sometimes followed by surgery and radiation therapies. All brought about by elevated PSA testing results. These included some patients whose PSA had gone up from below 2 to below 4 over the year and were then subjected to radiation treatment or surgery. Clearly, these men should have slotted into the active surveillance or watchful waiting categories. It also emphasizes the need for patients to become more aware of the various procedures and the attendant risks and benefits available to them. Also, it confirms the need for second opinions to be obtained.

In mid-2013, the American Urological Association (AUA) recommended that their members discontinue routine PSA testing for men in the age group 40 to 54 years old. Many doctors have no doubt heeded this call to limit PSA testing in this age group. There is a possibility that in the years ahead, many more men are going to present with prostate cancer that might be more advanced, than would have been the case under the past testing regime.

Access the USPSTF full report or a one page summary via Appendix 3. Access the AUA new PSA testing guidelines via Appendix 3.

Elimination of PSA testing would triple the number of men who have advanced prostate cancer at diagnosis, authors of a retrospective review concluded. *"Our analyses suggest that, if the pre-PSA era incidence rates were present in the modern U.S. population, then the total number of men presenting with M1 (metastatic) prostate cancer would be approximately three times greater than the number actually observed"* Edward M. Messing, MD, of the University of Rochester in New York, and co-authors, wrote in conclusion.[5]

It should be remembered that PSA testing and the DRE test are the basis of early prostate cancer diagnosis. The "over-servicing" by subsequent treatment is an issue best controlled by the patient and his medical professionals after careful consideration of ALL the facts and alternatives present.

Some men have significantly enlarged prostate glands brought about by benign prostate hypertrophy (BPH) or naturally. The average prostate size for a man aged 45 is around 40cc (cubic centimetres or millilitres). (My prostate at the time of diagnosis was considered small at 29cc – something of a let down to my manliness!). It is thought that with much larger prostates, the "normal safe" PSA level of 4 ng/ml, should be higher. Some doctors overlook this factor or are unaware of the benefit of calculating a **PSA Density** figure that takes into account the size of the prostate. The PSA density is a simple mathematical calculation derived from the division of the PSA value by prostate volume. The higher the PSA density, the greater is the likelihood of prostate cancer being present. A density of greater than 0.15 is more suggestive of prostate cancer. A density between 0.07 and 0.15 is in the grey area, with a density of under 0.07 is more suggestive of non-cancerous disease.[6]

If the DRE suggests to the doctor that you may have a prostate infection, or the lab analysis of your urine done at the same time as the PSA test shows an infection to be present, the PSA test should be repeated a few weeks later after the infection has been treated by a course of antibiotics. Similarly, should prostatitis (inflammation of the prostate gland) be present, a repeat PSA test should be done some weeks after the condition has been successfully treated.

It is also important to have your PSA sample sent to the same pathology lab on each occasion as there is often significant variance in results from lab to lab. My doctor provides me with a copy of the laboratory report after each PSA test which lists the results of the last 10 PSA results.

New and Future Developments in PSA Testing

Considerable research over the last decade has led to improvements in the PSA testing regime. One approach has been the development of new tests based on other tumour markers. Several newer blood tests seem to be more accurate than the PSA test, based on early studies. However, these tests are not yet in general use.

Another research development has focussed on an abnormal **gene** change found in prostate cells. This gene change in found in about half of all localized prostate cancer. It is rarely found in men without prostate cancer. This urine test should emerge into general use soon.

Many research studies, both of short or long duration, are underway. Prostate cancer is often a slow-growing cancer, so the effects of screening in these studies may become clearer in the coming years.

One genetic test that has reached the market in the USA and other countries including Australia et al., is the Progensa® **PCA3 test** marketed by Gen-Probe Inc. of San Diego, California. The PCA3-molecule was discovered some years ago, followed by the finding that concentrations of the PCA3 molecule are 100 times higher in prostate cancer cells than in normal prostate cells. In technical terms, this molecular assay detects the mRNA expression of the DD3 gene expressed in prostate cells. In recent studies, it was shown to have a specificity of 78% and a sensitivity of 57% in cancer vs. non-cancer. (By way of comparison, the PSA test, at modest elevations, has a specificity of as low as 20%, but rises to as much as 50% at levels ≥10 ng/ml).

As a result of a digital rectal examination (DRE), which includes the massaging of the prostate by the doctor, prostate cells, including potentially cancerous cells, are released into the urine. These cells can be detected in urine samples obtained after the DRE procedure is completed. This process is much less invasive for the patient than a prostate biopsy.

The PCA3 score is reported as a quantitative PCA3/PSA mRNA ratio x 1000 to normalize PCA3 to the amount of prostate RNA present in the urine sample. In cases, where insufficient PSA mRNA is present, are considered inconclusive. A score equal to or greater than 25 is considered positive. A positive result suggests an increased likelihood of a positive prostate cancer result being returned on biopsy.

In 2012, Beckman Coulter obtained FDA approval for their p2PSA blood test for PSA levels between 2 and 10 ng/ml. The test measures how much [-2]proPSA (a protein) is present in the blood. It determines the probability of having cancer using the [-2]proPSA measurement in conjunction with the total PSA and free PSA measurements from the same blood sample. The [-2]proPSA is a type of free PSA test and is associated with prostate cancer as higher levels of [-2]proPSA are found in the blood and tissue of prostate cancer patients. It is yet another tool in the growing arsenal of tests that provide the up-to-date medical practitioner, with better information on which to make a judgement call for or against a biopsy test at that time.

In the USA, we have seen a further development of the PCA3 diagnostic test into a three parameter test called **MiPS** or Mi-Prostate Score. The MiPS test is an early detection test (pre-biopsy) for prostate cancer that combines the amount of serum PSA, with the amounts of two genes in the urine. These two genes, TMPRSS2:ERG and PCA3, are specific for prostate cancer, meaning they are rarely present at high levels in the urine of men without prostate cancer. The MiPS combines serum PSA, urine TMPRSS2:ERG (also known as T2:ERG) and urine PCA3 to predict the likelihood of a patient having a positive prostate cancer determined by biopsy. The test also predicts the patient's risk of having potentially aggressive prostate cancer. The MiPS test was developed by the University of Michigan Health System and validated on almost 2,000 patients. The MiPS test is designed to help doctors and patients make a shared decision after

PSA testing about whether to monitor PSA levels or pursue a prostate biopsy. An interesting set of Questions and Answers on MiPS can be accessed via Appendix 3. This test presently costs US$731 in the USA.

Very recently, the FDA gave approval for the marketing of the Prostate Health Index or *phi* Test (Beckman Coulter) for patients with a PSA in the range 4 ng/ml to 10 ng/ml.[7] This test uses a mathematical formula that combines total PSA, free PSA, and p2PSA data to provide a Prostate Health Index level. In clinical trials among men with a standard PSA level between 2 and 10 ng/ml, the average (mean) *phi* scores were 34 for men who went on to have negative biopsies and 49 for men who went on to have positive biopsies, respectively. It is reasonably clear that in any large clinical study still to be done, that this test could be used to reduce the total number of patients for whom a biopsy is recommended. The present problem is how to interpret a *phi* test accurately in an individual patient. The results obtained only indicate a set of probabilities. The test would still provide false negatives and false positives. The test costs about $80 in the USA.

At the May 2014 American Urological Association meeting in Orlando, Dr Daniel Lin, MD, from the University of Washington in Seattle made a presentation on the newest test available, namely the **4K score test** (OPKO Diagnostics). The 4K score test was claimed to give a more accurate prediction of risk for a Gleason score of 7 or higher on biopsy than the PCPT calculator (version 2.0) (more on this calculator in the following chapter).[8] The 4K score blood test is an assay panel that combines three PSA measures (total, free, and intact) with another prostate-specific measure, **human kallikrein 2 (hK2)**, in an algorithm that takes into account a patient's age, digital rectal exam result, and previous biopsy status. The test costs about $395 in the USA. The test offers the same limitations as the *phi* test, when the result is considered for an individual patient. False positives and negatives are likely in some instances, which make a precise decision as to whether to biopsy or not to biopsy, harder. However, it might be possible to consider having two standard PSA tests done (the second a couple of months after the first), and then a *phi* test followed by a 4K score test. The two PSA test results, together with the other patient metrics, provide a cancer risk assessment on the

PCPT calculator. Should all four values suggest a likelihood of a Gleason score of 7 or higher being found on biopsy, it is a pretty clear case to have a 10 core (or greater) biopsy as soon as possible.

Other Genetic Testing

At the European Society for Radiotherapy and Oncology (ESTRO) 33rd annual conference held in early 2014 in Vienna, Dr Robert Bristow, MD, PhD., a senior scientist at the Ontario Cancer Institute and professor of medical biophysics at the University of Toronto, in Canada, reported on a new genetic test that his group was developing. This DNA test, based on the type of genetic signature found, could see patients having an intensified treatment regime, which might not have been suggested based on the Gleason Score and other clinical parameters. Similarly, the absence of the genetic signature, could allow patients to be treated less aggressively than might have been suggested by the patient's clinical parameters. Should this test finally reach the market (as seems likely), it will be the first such genetic test that can help frame the initial treatment protocols. The other genetic tests available are based on RNA analysis of sample tissue taken from removed prostate gland.[9]

Mutations in BRCA1 and BRCA2 genes were originally spotted some years ago in women with breast cancer. More recent research has confirmed that these faulty genes not only raise the risk of developing breast cancer, but also of ovarian and prostate cancers. The results of a major study in the May 2013 Journal of Clinical Oncology, reported that 1.2% of men with prostate cancer carry the BRCA2 mutation and 0.44% have the BRCA1 mutation. Carrying the BRCA2 mutation gives a man an 8.6 times higher risk of developing prostate cancer compared to a non-carrier. If a man carries the BRCA1 mutation, he has a 3.4-fold higher risk. The BRCA2-prostate cancers that arise in these men also tend to be more aggressive.[10] You should discuss genetic testing with your doctors, if there is a family history of breast and prostate cancer.

Biopsy Testing

If your prostate specific antigen (PSA) test or digital rectal exam (DRE) is abnormal, doctors may do more tests to diagnose prostate cancer. These are likely to include:

A transrectal ultrasound (TRUS): A probe the size of a finger is inserted into the rectum, and high-energy sound waves (ultrasound) are bounced off the prostate to create a picture of the prostate, called a sonogram. The sonogram indicates the shape and nature of the prostate. It does not detect cancer. The ultrasound is used to ensure that samples are taken reliably from different parts of the prostate. It might also identify areas of the prostate that appear 'suspicious" or areas determined as abnormal by DRE.

Biopsy: A series of small pieces of tissue are removed from the prostate and examined under a microscope by a pathologist to see if there are cancer cells present in the prostate tissue samples. There are generally three types of protocols used for undertaking a biopsy. These all relate to the comfort of the patient whilst the prostate tissue is obtained. Biopsy tests without sedation appear to be less common today, due to the higher number of biopsy (rods) samples taken. The taking of samples can be somewhat daunting for the patient, particularly if the urologist doesn't have an assistant to log and identify the position of each sample taken. Under these circumstances, it could take up to 30 minutes or more for the biopsy samples to be taken and logged with the sampling probe perhaps removed a number of times and re-inserted.

Some urologists use local anaesthetics around the prostate to increase patient comfort. Today the majority of urologists do the biopsy under a general anaesthetic. After the patient is "put under", the urologist uses the ultrasound probe to produce a sonogram that allows him/her to guide the insertion of a small spring-loaded needle through the rectal wall into the prostate. Usually between 12 to as many as 24 tissue samples (often referred to as cores) are taken from the prostate during an initial first biopsy. These cores are usually about the thickness of a toothpick and about 10mm long. Some urologists still only take 6 to 10 tissue samples which can increase the chance of missing the cancerous areas of the prostate.

It is now possible to carry out "targeted" biopsies under MRI. The cost of MRI-based biopsies is higher than that of TRUS-guided biopsies. This type of biopsy is increasing in popularity, but is not widely used as yet, mainly due to urologists being committed to well-practised techniques, the time taken to complete the procedure and the lack of 3 Tesla field strength MRI machines, which give the best results. See the following section for more details on a MRI-based biopsy.

Prior to a prostate biopsy, patients should make sure that their urologist is advised of all medications that they are normally taking on a day-to-day basis. Patients who take aspirin, warfarin, or clopidogrel (Plavix®) — or other so-called "blood thinners" — are normally asked to stop taking such drugs for a period of time prior to a biopsy procedure, and should discuss the appropriate time to stop taking such drugs (and when to restart them after biopsy) with their primary care physician or their cardiologist, as appropriate. I suffer from atrial fibrillation, and take Warfarin daily to prevent blood clotting. My cardiologist prescribed Clexane® as a substitute for the daily Warfarin dose in the lead up to and immediately following the biopsy. My wife enjoyed the twice daily injections into my abdomen area!

If the urologist believes that the cancer may be present in the front part of the prostate, the biopsies may be taken using a different technique, which is called the Perineal Method. This involves taking sample rods from the prostate via the area between the anus and the scrotum, which is called the perineum.

There are instances, where cancer is not detected via the first biopsy, due to low level cancer. A negative biopsy is not completely conclusive that cancer is not present. The patient's PSA is usually monitored on a regular basis (probably 6 monthly) after a negative biopsy result. An increasing PSA result, may lead to a second series of biopsies being undertaken.

Use of a general anaesthetic dictates that the procedure is undertaken in a day clinic or hospital with a patient being discharged a few hours after the procedure is completed. Some urologists undertake the procedure with patients under sedation or local anaesthetic in their specialist rooms. The urologist will prescribe a course of antibiotics to be started before and after the procedure to lessen the chance of infection. Post the procedure, the patient is likely to experience some rectal bleeding, blood in the urine and blood staining of the ejaculate. Blood in the ejaculate should cease over the following few weeks.

Magnetic Resonance Imaging and biopsies – A quantum leap forward in technology?

Most of us have had an MRI at one time or other. If you have had one you will certainly remember it, as it's a very loud machine! It's also somewhat claustrophobic as you are inserted into a smallish tunnel (smaller than that in a CT scan) and sometimes have a head guard fitted. Music is often provided to deaden the noise emitted from the machine as it collects your image, slice by slice. Of course, patients with metallic implants and pacemakers are not generally able to have MRI scans.

Considerable research into the use of variances of Magnetic Resonance Imaging (MRI) to assist in the detection and assessment of prostate cancer has been ongoing for at least fifteen years. The development and introduction of these advances has manifested itself in the form of **multiparametric MRI (mpMRI).**

MRI machines have been commercially available since about 1982 when General Electric introduced the first whole body scanner with a magnet of 1.5 Tesla field strength. Some 20,000 of these 1.5 Tesla machines have been in daily use in hospitals and clinics in practically every country on earth. The introduction of the higher strength and higher resolution 3 Tesla systems, a few years ago, together with accessories specifically suited to tumour detection and biopsy sampling are revolutionizing prostate cancer detection and quantitation. The high field strength and associated magnetic "gradients" of 3T machines, allow the collection of tumour specific information for tumours as small as 0.5 ml in volume. The machine can be set up to detect high-grade clinically significant prostate cancer rather than low-grade disease that does not require active management.

It is usual for a gadolinium-based contrasting agent to be intravenously injected before the MRI session begins. The newer systems generally complete the scan in lesser time than the earlier machines which often went on for 40 to 60 minutes.

Should the scan reveal the presence of tumours, it is possible (but unlikely) for the interventional radiologist to collect biopsy samples from each tumour of size, during the MRI session. This is referred to as a direct "in-bore" biopsy. Of course, non-magnetic needles are required to complete this sampling. This procedure replaces the TRUS procedure and it gives greater certainty that no significant cancerous lesion has been missed, even in hard to get to areas of the prostate.

A second procedure, called a fusion biopsy, sees the use of a device that "fuses" the stored MRI image with real-time ultrasound images. This technique is rapidly increasing in popularity.

The Wesley Hospital in Brisbane, Australia, recently concluded a two-year study[11] which showed that their mpMRI approach to diagnosing prostate cancer is highly effective in identifying life-threatening prostate cancer and at the same time reduces over-diagnosis of non-life-threatening prostate cancer. The study found that the use of multiparametric MRI (mpMRI):

Reduced the number of men needing prostate biopsies by 51%.

Reduced the problem of over-diagnosis of non-life threatening disease by about 90%.

Had 92% sensitivity in diagnosing life-threatening prostate cancer. (Compared with the TRUS method for prostate cancer diagnosis which had 70% sensitivity in diagnosing life-threatening prostate cancer).

Multiparametric MRI (mpMRI) is so-called due to a host of software and accessories that substantially extend its clinical use. The following techniques are now in widespread use to help differentiate between malignant and benign tissue within the prostate:

T2-Weighted (T2W) imaging

In this mode the image contrast is weighted to demonstrate different anatomical structures or pathologies. It provides high resolution images of the anatomy of the prostate and its capsular wall.

Diffusion-weighted imaging (DW-MRI)

It determines the Brownian motion of free water within tissue. The increased cellularity and lesser extracellular spaces found in cancer lesions are detectable as regions of restricted diffusion by DW-MRI. The image obtained shows a contrast between diseased and healthy tissue. The impedance of water molecules diffusion can be quantitatively assessed using the apparent diffusion coefficient (ADC) value, and yields a different, but complementary image to DW imaging. The ADC value is automatically calculated by the system software.

Dynamic contrast enhanced MRI (DCE-MRI)

It records in real time the vascularity of tumours by the distribution of the wash-in or wash-out of the gadolinium contrasting agent between tissue and the blood pool. This allows the characterization of alterations in the microvascular environment resulting from tumour **angiogenesis**. Higher grade and large tumours are detected due to their tendency to have higher wash-in and wash-out rates. Lower grade smaller tumours are often not detected by DCE-MRI.

MR spectroscopy

It examines the concentration of biochemical disease markers, such as citrate, choline and creatinine, in tissues. Healthy prostate tissue has low level of choline and high levels of citrate, whereas cancerous prostate tissue, display the converse, i.e. high choline and lower citrate levels.

Access more information on mpMRI via Appendix 3. Alternatively, review the paper titled *Advancements in MR Imaging of the Prostate: From Diagnosis to Interventions* by David Bonekamp, et al., published in the journal RadioGraphics.[12]

As we have read earlier, prostate cancer is diagnosed by a pathologist histologically examining biopsy samples that have been (mainly) obtained using a transrectal ultrasonic-guided device. Sampling error could cause cancerous growths to be missed and indolent cancers are often over-detected leading to unnecessary clinical intervention. The recent introduction of more powerful (and thus higher resolution) MRI systems has seen mpMRI come to the fore as a prostate cancer diagnostic tool. [13]

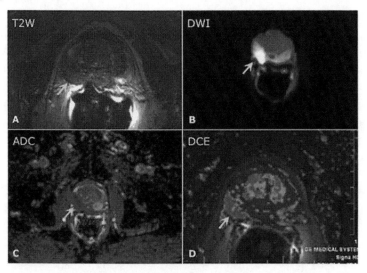

Image: Courtesy of Radiology Rounds Vol. 8, Issue 8, 2010 newsletter

The Axial Multiparametric MR Images above are: A) T2-weighted, B) diffusion weighted (DWI), C) apparent diffusion coefficient (ADC) and D) dynamic contrast enhanced (DCE) images of a patient with prostate cancer. The tumour appears dark on the axial T2-weighted image (arrow); the corresponding area shows restricted diffusion on the DWI and ADC images as well as abnormal contrast enhancement on the DCE axial image (as evident from abnormal red colour coding of the tumour).

A new prostate-imaging technology that fuses MRI with real-time three-dimensional ultrasound may offer a more exacting method to obtain biopsy specimens from suspicious areas within the organ. This 2011 development at UCLA combines the use of an MRI with advanced Doppler ultrasound technology to produce a 3D "fusion" image that is used to accurately target "suspicious" areas of the prostate. The MRI-ultrasound fusion technique is best suited to those who have had prior negative biopsies, but have persistently elevated PSA levels, and for "active surveillance" patients (those with low-risk prostate cancers, who are being carefully monitored over time to see if their cancer progresses or becomes more aggressive). The UCLA team found that targeted biopsy was about five times more likely to find cancer than non-targeted, systematic biopsy. More details and a video on the technique are accessed via Appendix 3.

The use of an endorectal coil (ERC) provides higher accuracy than other modalities in assessing seminal vesicle invasion and extra-capsular extension (ECE) of prostate cancer (96% and 81% respectively). Another study found the ERC provided an overall sensitivity and specificity for ECE of 75 % and 92 %, respectively.[14]

The importance of mpMRI as a diagnostic tool for prostate cancer was emphasised in early 2012 when the European Society of Urogenital Radiology introduced their ESUR prostate MR Guidelines.[15] These clinical guidelines for the multi-parametric MRI of the prostate were prepared by a group of prostate MRI experts from the ESUR, and are based on literature evidence and consensus expert opinion. The guidelines outline the optimal technique recommended for prostate cancer diagnosis and include three protocols for the "detection" of prostate cancer, the "staging" of the disease and, in the case of metastatic cancer, the "node and bone" progression of the disease. They also cover the use of an endorectal coil to improve signal to noise ratios (resolution) and compare the endorectal coil verses the alternative non-invasive pelvic phased-array coil. It also reviews the difference in performance of the earlier 1.5 Tesla systems verses the more sensitive 3 T machines.

A new scoring system, called the PI-RADS classification system, to enable uniform structured reporting of prostate cancer mpMRI results, is postulated. PI-RADS is an abbreviation for Prostate Imaging Reporting and Data System and is broadly based on the breast cancer scoring system, BI-RADS.

Not all MRI facilities use all three of TW2, DW, and DCE, with even fewer using the Spectroscopy capability. PI-RADS assists in the 'standardisation' of result reporting in these instances. It also provides scoring that can be linked back to the universal Gleason scoring system.[16]

Staging - A Positive Biopsy Result

The tissue removed during the biopsy is examined by a pathologist under the microscope to look for abnormal or cancerous cells in the tissue. If cancer cells are present the pathologist will grade the tumour/s against an internationally accepted scale for grading prostate cancer, called the **Gleason Score**.

Gleason scores range from 2 to 10. Tumours with higher grades tend to grow faster than those with lower grades and they are also more likely to spread. Doctors use tumour grade along with your age and other factors to suggest treatment options. To determine the Gleason score, the pathologist examines the patterns of cells in the prostate tissue samples. The most common pattern of cells is given a grade of 1 - this being most like normal prostate tissue - to grade 5 (most abnormal). The pathologist gives the second most common pattern a grade of 1 to 5 and then adds the grades for the two most common patterns together to make the Gleason score (3 + 4 = 7). If only one pattern is seen, the pathologist counts it twice (5 + 5 = 10). Gleason grades of 6 or less suggest a low risk from the cancer. A score of 7 suggests moderately differentiated cells and an intermediate risk. Scores of 8 to 10 suggest high risk to the patient. A high Gleason score (such as 10) means a high-grade prostate tumour.

See image on the next page.

Staging – TNM Score

Doctors also provide a different score which records how far the cancer has spread. The **TNM Score** is used around the world to stage cancers which develop as tumours and metastasise elsewhere in the body. The letters T, N and M refer to different locations of the cancer.

(In the United States, a different system is still in use which uses Roman numerals. A Stage I cancer is early stage cancer whereas a Stage IV cancer has spread to other parts of the body).

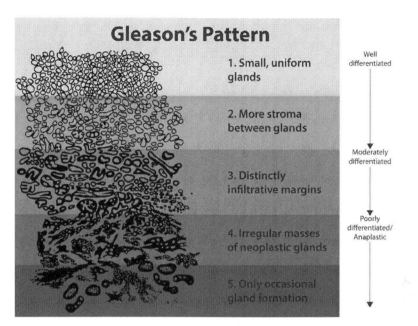

Image: SEER Training Modules, *Prostate Cancer*. U. S. National Institutes of Health, National Cancer Institute. 1st February. 2015 http://training.seer.cancer.gov/prostate/abstract-code-stage/morphology.html/>.

The **T score** is the rating and size of the primary tumour. **T1** tumours cannot be felt by DRE or by imaging. Cancer is on occasion found in biopsy samples taken when a patient undergoes a surgical procedure for an enlarged prostate. This phenomenum is often referred to as an incidental finding. In these occurrences, the T1 score is further recorded as T1a, T1b or T1c with T1a and T1b referring to the incidental findings. T1c tumours are ones found by needle biopsy.

T2 tumours can be felt by doctors during DRE. They also may be seen with an **imaging test**. T2 tumours are those that haven't grown outside the prostate and are based on cancer growth within the left or right lobes of the prostate. T2a tumours haven't grown beyond half of one lobe. T2b have grown beyond half of one lobe. T2c tumours have grown in both lobes.

T3 tumours have grown outside the prostate. They have reached the **seminal vesicles**, the neck of the bladder, or the connective tissue around the prostate. Imaging tests are used to locate T3 and T4 tumours. **T4** tumours have spread to tissue near the prostate including the external sphincter, rectum, bladder levator muscles and pelvic wall.

Staging – Nodes

The **N** category indicates if the cancer has spread to the nearby lymph nodes. Imaging tests determine these values. **N0** means that the cancer has not spread to the lymph nodes. **N1** means it has spread into the nearby lymphatic system. **NX** means it is unknown if the cancer has reached the lymph nodes.

Staging – Metastasis

The **M** score indicates that the cancer has spread to distant body sites which include other lymph nodes, the bones or liver. It is only determined after at least two imaging tests.

M scores for prostate cancer include:

MX – unknown if cancer has spread to distant sites

M0 – no growth in distant sites

M1 – cancer has spread to distant sites

M1a – cancer that has spread to lymph nodes

M1b – cancer that has spread to bones

M1c – cancer that has spread to distant organs.

Imaging Tests

Before the doctors determine a course of action to treat localised or advanced prostate cancer, it is necessary for the patient to undergo a Bone Scan and a CT Scan (or an MRI Scan instead of the CT Scan). These tests might determine whether or not, the cancer has spread to the lymph nodes, the seminal vesicles, other organs or the bones **(metastasis).**

Bone Scan

The purpose of the bone scan is to see if the cancer has spread to the bones. It is done on a PET machine. (PET stands for Positron Emission

Tomography). A small amount of low dose radioactive material (usually technetium) is injected in an arm vein. The test, which requires the patient to lie still on a padded table for about 40 minutes, is started about two hours after the technetium is injected. The padded table is introduced below a special (gamma) camera that "sees" the radioactive material. Prostate cancer, reaching the pelvic bone or spine, causes damage to the bones. The efforts of the bone to repair itself attract the radioactive material and these areas appear as "hot spots" on the bone scan.

Other medical conditions can also lead to the concentration of the radioactive material in the areas of bone repair. The radiologist is proficient in determining what prostate cancer is and what is not. Of course, if the cancer has only just migrated to the bones, insufficient cancer cells may be present to have caused bone damage. A bone scan is rarely positive when the PSA level is less than 20 ng/ml. If the bone scan determines that the cancer has spread to the bones, it will be necessary for the patient to undertake treatments that target whole body cancer.

Test results are usually only available about 48 hours after the test is completed. Patients undergoing a bone scan can resume normal activities after the scan has been completed. (Some patients are given a sedative before the scan to assist them to remain still whilst undertaking the test. This sedative needs to wear off before normal activities, like driving a car, are resumed).

CT Scan or MRI Scan

A CT or CAT scan refers to a **computerised tomography** scan, is a simple and routine test that takes up to an hour. Dye is injected into an arm vein and the patient also drinks a fluid that helps contrast images of the pelvic area. The purpose of the CT scan is to provide information of the possible spread of the cancer to the lymph nodes in the pelvic area. It also provides very accurate measurement of the size and precise position of the prostate relative to the surrounding organs. These measurements are very important for the planning of any **external beam radiation** that might follow these imaging tests.

Magnetic Resonance Imaging (MRI) uses a powerful magnetic field to produce pictures of the internal organs, bone and soft body tissue to again determine if the cancer has spread outside of the prostate. A MRI is a more claustrophobic and noisy test than a CT scan. Patients are required to remove all metallic objects such as watches and jewellery before undergoing a MRI. The MRI images produced also assist in planning for future prostate **surgery**.

It is possible that the CT or MRI scan will detect the spread of the cancer to the lymph nodes near the prostate gland. In these cases, it is likely that the patient will be required to pay a return visit for a further CT or MRI scan, during which a fine needle aspiration procedure will be undertaken under local anaesthetic. This procedure provides a biopsy sample from the lymph nodes for pathological analysis. We will hear a lot more about MRI elsewhere in the book.

Colour Doppler Ultrasound

We learnt earlier that a transrectal ultrasound (TRUS) is a non-invasive procedure in which an ultrasonic probe is inserted into the rectum in order to take an image of the prostate. It works by using a technique called the **Doppler Effect**. It allows the doctor to "see" the prostate and accurately determine its volume and dimensions. The volume of the prostate is used to calculate a predicted PSA value. This value is compared with the patient's actual PSA value with higher actual values signalling further possible testing and intervention. Men with very large prostates usually have a higher "normal" PSA value than those with prostates that are of average size. It is also used in the biopsy procedure. Most urologists use systems that provide black and white images only. In recent years, the Colour Doppler Ultrasound system has been favoured over the black and white version, as it offers higher resolution, greater precision and includes tissue harmonic technology. There is also another higher sensitivity version of the Colour Doppler which is the Power Colour Doppler Ultrasound. The Power Doppler is often referred to as the Energy Doppler, as it operates by measuring the power (energy) of the many different frequency shifts inside each measurement cell, which are added to form the power signal. The very latest Colour Doppler machines offer sensitivities similar to or even better than the Power Doppler Ultrasound machines.

The most important consideration for using a Colour Doppler TRUS, is its ability to more accurately detect small abnormalities within the prostate by observing its blood flow patterns. If higher blood flows are detected, it is likely that the indicated areas are cancerous, due to **neovascularity** (abundance of blood vessels inside the tumour). In cases, where the PSA level is higher than the predicted level and anomalous areas are detected, it would be appropriate for a biopsy to be undertaken. The absence of these two factors would suggest a follow up PSA down the track and a watchful waiting stance be adopted.

The recently-developed Tissue Harmonic technology, referred to above, improves spatial resolution of the system to permit visualization of smaller objects and improves contrast resolution to provide very subtle differences in the grayscale of the Doppler image. The technique of using Tissue Harmonic technology with Colour Doppler TRUS practiced by Dr. Duke Bahn of the Prostate Institute of America, also evaluates the likelihood of the prostate cancer being fully confined to the prostate or otherwise. Access full details of his procedure via Appendix 3. He also suggests that further improvements in Colour Doppler TRUS technology are imminent, which might further enhance its usefulness. Thus, Power and Colour Doppler Ultrasound are very important tools in the pre-diagnosis of prostate cancer before biopsy. Together with mpMRI, these techniques are likely to lead to fewer unnecessary biopsies being undertaken and random biopsies being passed into history in favour of the targeted biopsy. In coming years, it should become common practice for men with elevated PSA levels to undergo both these procedures before a biopsy is recommended.

Patient Indices

The completion of questionnaires by patients assists urologists in their pre and post-treatment options. These reveal some or all of the following indices or scores:

The International Prostate Symptom Score (IPSS), International Index of Erectile Function-15 (IIEF-15), UCLA-Expanded Prostate Cancer Index Composite (EPIC), and the Functional Assessment of Cancer Therapy-Prostate (FACT-P) score.

The International Prostate Symptom Score (IPSS) is an 8 question (7 symptom questions + 1 quality of life question) in the form of a questionnaire, with the answers used to screen for, rapidly diagnose, track the symptoms of, and suggest management of the symptoms of the disease benign prostatic hyperplasia (BPH). The IPSS is designed for easy completion by the patient and assists the medical practitioner in formulating treatment for the condition. It was designed by the American Urological Association in the 90's and it originally lacked the 8th quality of life question, hence its original name: the American Urological Association symptom score (AUA-7).

International Index of Erectile Function-15 (IIEF-15) is a brief 15-item, self-administered questionnaire that was developed as a measure to detect treatment-related erectile function in patients in cross-cultural settings. Relevant cross-cultural domains of sexual function were identified via the literature and were reviewed and endorsed by an international panel of experts. These include: Erectile Function (6 items), Orgasmic Function (2 items), Sexual Desire (2 items), Intercourse Satisfaction (3 items) and Overall Satisfaction (2 items). The 15 questions are answered by the patient against provided criteria with the results of considerable use to the urologist.

Expanded Prostate Cancer Index Composite (EPIC) is a questionnaire that requests the patient to quantify against provided criteria, levels of urinary function, bowel activities, sexual function and overall satisfaction post treatment.

Functional Assessment of Cancer Therapy-Prostate (FACT-P) is a multidimensional, self-report Quality of Life questionnaire specifically designed for use with prostate cancer patients. It consists of 27 core items which assess patient function in four areas: Physical, Social/Family, Emotional, and Functional well-being, and is further supplemented by 12 site specific items to assess for prostate related symptoms.

The PCPT Prostate Cancer Risk Calculator was the first on-line prostate cancer risk assessment tool to allow men to assess their own risk for prostate cancer. This calculator emerged from the Prostate Cancer Prevention Trial (PCPT) in the USA. Obviously, the results obtained *should always be discussed with your doctor*. The tool developed in 2006 by Thompson, et al., is based on data developed from 5,519 men in the placebo group of the PCPT trial. It exclusively included men who went on to have a biopsy after the completion of the therapy stage of the trial. The tool was upgraded in 2012 after further patient data came available from the PCPT trial. This improved calculator is referred to as the PCPTRC2.0. It is accessible via Appendix 3. Their **nomogram** is based on: PSA result, DRE findings, any prior biopsy data, age, family history of prostate cancer, and ethnicity. It is still considered to be **the** nomogram for assessment of the risk for prostate cancer, even though newer nomograms, such as the Sunnybrook nomogram, which assess additional data, have arrived on the scene. Let's look at an example using my data:

Age: **68 years**

PSA level: **7.5 ng/ml**

Ethnic background: **Caucasian**

Family history of prostate cancer: **Yes (Father and Brother)**

Positive or negative DRE result: **Negative**

Prior negative prostate biopsy: **None**

With this data inserted into the PCPT calculator, the results are:

Estimated risk of biopsy-detectable high-risk prostate cancer: **13 percent**

Estimated risk of biopsy-detectable low-risk prostate cancer: **26 percent**

Probability of a negative biopsy result (i.e., no evidence of prostate cancer): **61 percent**

Chance that he will have an infection that *may* require hospitalization: **2 to 4 percent.**

Clearly, the results from the calculator can only be considered a guide and the results obtained must be discussed with your doctor. Let's put my actual results into perspective against the above results:

Diagnosed with intermediate prostate cancer with a Gleason Score of 3+4 = 7

Nine out of 24 biopsy cores were positive for cancer.

The University of Texas Health System Centre web site also includes an updated version of the calculator that allows any PCA3 test data to be added if you have had this test.

The **Sunnybrook Prostate Cancer Risk Calculator** uses the same criteria as the PCPTRC2.0 calculator plus the patient's urinary symptoms (measured by the International Prostate Symptom Score index) and the Free to Total PSA ratio value. Unfortunately, I don't have the results of these two values available and as such cannot compare the two calculator results. The Sunnybrook calculator is accessible via Appendix 3. (Sunnybrook Health Sciences Centre, Toronto, Canada). Both hospital web sites include a video on the use of their calculator as well as requiring persons wanting to use the calculators to acknowledge a disclaimer before accessing the calculator.

PART 2: TREATMENT OPTIONS

Chapter 4.
Introductory Comments on Treatment Options

So you are diagnosed with prostate cancer. The urologist will discuss at length the nature of your disease, the treatment options available to you, and how the treatment options might match your priorities. Sometimes the most aggressive and effective treatment causes side effects that the patient might not be able to accept or cope with. You will be informed of the extent of your prostate cancer (**stage**) and the rate at which it is growing (**grade**).

It is a good idea to have your wife or other confidant, also attend this interview with the specialist, as it is very difficult for the patient to remain psychologically composed enough to taken in all the information imparted by the specialist. It is also appropriate to make a list of questions to ask the specialist and take the list with you to the appointment. Don't be embarrassed by the nature of your questions. Remember it's the specialist's responsibility to fully inform you as regards your condition, the threat it might pose to your health, the possible treatment options and the relevant side effects. Also bear in mind that prostate cancer is generally a slow progression disease. It is thus appropriate that time be taken to make a decision on the most appropriate treatment for you. This is likely to require you to make a return visit to your specialist some days or weeks after you have been informed of your PC diagnosis. This is particularly relevant for men diagnosed with localised prostate cancer. It is likely that the specialist will provide you with hardcopy material of treatment options, side effects etc. when you are informed that you have prostate cancer. Study these carefully to get a better understanding of the treatment options, side effects, and risks to your health, etc.

It is likely that the specialist will also discuss with you the impact of your age, and other health conditions that you might have, on the treatment proposed. Life expectancy, of say, a 55 year old male is quite different to an 80 year old man who might have other serious health conditions which suggest a life expectancy of less than the average life expectancy of around 8 years. The doctor may refer to nonograms, which are prediction tools that can be used to decide which treatment approaches will result in the greatest benefit for men at various stages of prostate cancer.

A pre-treatment (post biopsy) nomogram can be used to predict the probability of cancer remaining progression-free following radical prostatectomy or brachytherapy. The nomogram lists the latest patient data versus the doctor's or institution "standard" criteria:

Most recent PSA (prostate-specific antigen) value.

Primary and secondary Gleason grade.

Doctor's assessment of patient's clinical tumour stage (TNM details).

Number of positive cores (samples) found during biopsy.

Number of negative cores (samples) found during biopsy.

Planned radiation therapy dose if patient has already seen a radiation oncologist.

Whether patient has had previous treatment with hormones.

Whether patient has had radiation treatment.

Jani and Hellman in 2003 reported (Lancet 361 1045-1053) the increasing complication rates for early stage prostate cancer suffers are as shown in the table on the next page[1]:

Issue	Prostatectiomy	EBRT	Brachytherapy	Brachytherapy with EBRT
Rectal	+	+++	+	++
Impotence	+++	++	+	++
Incontinence	+++	+	+	+
Urine Retention	+	+	+++	+++

Increasing number of +s indicates increasing complication rates

The following are the **ten main treatment options**, some of which have different subsets that provide considerably different outcomes:

Watchful Waiting or Active Surveillance

Surgery

Radiation Therapy

-External Beam Radiation Therapy (EBRT)

-3-D CRT, IMRT, IGRT and Tomography

-Stereotactic Body Radiotherapy (SBRT)

-Proton Beam Therapy (PBT)

-Low Dose Brachytherapy (Seeds)

-High Dose Brachytherapy plus X-Ray Radiation

Hyperthermia

Cryotherapy

High Intensity Focussed Ultrasound (HIFU)

Focal Laser Ablation (FLA)

Hormone Therapy

Chemotherapy and Immunotherapy

Complementary and Alternative Therapies

We look at these in appropriate detail in Chapters 5 to 14 that follow. At the end of each of these chapters, a summary of the treatment is outlined in easily-understood language and a partial set of pros and cons for and against the treatment are listed.

Chapter 5.
Active Surveillance (or Watchful Waiting)

Active Surveillance and Watchful Waiting are often regarded as being the same. Sometimes the term 'Observation or Observational Management' is also used.

Watchful Waiting - the urologist may advise that treatment is not required. This is more usual for men over 70 with a slow-growing cancer. However, it is important for PSA levels to be regularly monitored and a DRE be done to check for any abnormalities that might develop. Older patients with slow-growing low grade cancer are more likely to die of a cause other than prostate cancer. If the PSA levels starts to elevate or irregularities are found after a DRE, it is likely that one of a number of interventions will be prescribed.

Active Surveillance - no standardised definition for Active Surveillance appears to exist. One study of 16 cohorts used different monitoring protocols, all with different combinations for DRE, PSA, re-biopsy and/or imaging findings. These different protocols also appeared to present differences in curative and palliative treatment objectives.[1] Active surveillance is an appropriate option for men with low volume, low risk prostate cancer. This approach maintains quality of life and provides excellent cancer survival rates. Currently, candidates for active surveillance (including watchful waiting) constitute approximately half of all men with newly diagnosed prostate cancer.

The US National Comprehensive Cancer Network (NCCN) has recently updated their Prostate Cancer Guidelines™. These Guidelines attempt to standardise Active Surveillance protocols for low grade and intermediate risk prostate cancer sufferers. It is a most comprehensive 92 page essay on prostate cancer which is well worth viewing. Access it via Appendix 3.

"There are several variables that must be considered in order to tailor prostate cancer therapy to an individual patient and the NCCN Guidelines provide a solid framework on which to base these

treatment discussions and subsequent decisions," said Dr James L. Mohler, who is the chairman of the NCCN Guidelines Panel for Prostate Cancer. *"The current NCCN Guidelines recommend that at age 40, high-risk men begin annual PSA and DRE. All other men at age 40 should be offered a baseline PSA and DRE and if their PSA is 1.0 ng/ml or greater, they should receive annual follow-ups. If their PSA is less than 1.0, the NCCN Guidelines recommend that these men be early detected again at age 45,"* said Dr Mohler.[2]

The NCCN Guidelines have established a new "very low risk" category that incorporates the strictest Epstein criteria from all definitions for clinically insignificant prostate cancer. In addition, active surveillance and only active surveillance is now the recommendation for many men diagnosed with prostate cancer. Men with low risk prostate cancer who have a life expectancy of less than 10 years and men with very low risk prostate cancer with a life expectancy of less than 20 years should be offered and recommended active surveillance.

Findings from a Canadian study of 452 men by Klotz, et al., suggest that the 10 year actuarial survival rate of low grade prostate cancer on an active surveillance protocol was 97.2%.[3] What constitutes an active surveillance protocol? The **Epstein criteria** of **clinically insignificant prostate cancer** (CIPC) are the most widely used by urology professionals. It suggested parameters are: clinical stage T2 or less, Gleason Score of 6 or lower, PSA density 0.15 ng/ml or lower, and less than 33% positive cores on biopsy.[4,5]

It should be noted that C. Jeldres, et al., in a paper in the European Urologist in December 2009, found that the Epstein criteria may understate the true nature of prostate cancer in European men by as much as 25%. Thus, it cautions the use of the Epstein criteria as the sole basis for a treatment regime.[6]

Another paper on the web site of the Prostate Cancer Research Institute in the USA by Professor Laurence Klotz, Professor of Surgery, University of Toronto, is a most informative examination of matters pertaining to low risk (< Gleason 7) patients. This paper also thoroughly covers the issue of the rapid **PSA doubling time (PSADT)** which is a very important parameter in judging the degree of aggressiveness of the cancer. Access this paper via Appendix 3.

A search of published scientific papers suggests the following parameters for a candidate for active surveillance:

Generally 55 year old or younger with a PSA level of <10 ng/ml; with a Gleason Score of 6 or less; and TNM value of T1c or T2a (with one tumour of less than 50% of one lobe); 25% or less of cores positive for cancer; with a PSA density of less than 0.15. For men older than 55, the PSA level might be 10 – 12 ng/ml or slightly higher for men in their seventies.

The April 2014 Prostate Cancer Guidelines of the European Urology Association suggest the following parameters for active surveillance candidates: *over 10 years of life-expectancy, cT1-2, PSA ≤ 10 ng/ml, biopsy Gleason score ≤ 6 (at least 10 cores), ≤ 2 positive biopsies, minimal biopsy core involvement (≤ 50% cancer per biopsy).*[7]

It is essential that you get specific advice from your medical team as regards your possible suitability to go on an active surveillance program. Urologists universally agree that it is very important for men adhering to an active surveillance regimen, to make a strict commitment to regular PSA and DRE testing AND an annual or two-yearly biopsy. The PSA and DRE should be done quarterly in the first year, followed by six monthly tests thereafter assuming that results stay within limits acceptable to your medical practitioner. Should there be an adverse change in your results, the medical practitioner is likely to call for active intervention. It is probable that around 30% of active surveillance patients will require active intervention within a 5 year period of initial cancer diagnosis.

To put things into perspective, research by Dr Sung Kyu Hong, et al., from the Seoul National University Bundang Hospital [8] has shown that the clinical and biopsy-related parameters currently available, have limited value in the prediction of pathologically insignificant or unfavourable prostate cancer in patents with a single positive core and low PSA level. Further efforts are and should be made to identify more accurate predictors of actual pathological characteristics and/or prognoses of prostate cancers to improve the selection of candidates for active surveillance or alternatively active intervention.

The **"Cancer Anxiety Factor"** is a powerful psychological circumstance that afflicts all men when told that they have prostate cancer. Many feel that they have to take positive action to rid their body of this treacherous and often fatal disease. Unfortunately, many urologists with the best of intent, advise their patients to undertake active intervention, which plays right into the patient's frame of mind of wishing to be free of the threat. Institutions and most urologists in private practice recognise the patient's vulnerability at that time and provide psychosocial support that might assist the patient to make a decision to join an active surveillance program. Most prostate cancers diagnosed today are Stage T1c, suggesting the biopsy was undertaken purely on the basis of an elevated PSA and no DRE abnormality. While many threatening cancers are detected at this stage (T1c), over-treatment of T1c prostate cancers is now a concern to medical administrators.

Summary – Active Surveillance and Watchful Waiting

There is often confusion in the exact meaning of these two terms. A consensus for watchful waiting probably suggests less testing and intervention than in active surveillance and more reliance on changes in a man's symptoms to trigger a medical response. Active surveillance calls for a specific and regular testing regime including a DRE, PSA testing and in some instances, a biopsy and even imaging.

More than half of all men diagnosed with low risk disease conform well to an active surveillance regime.

Various international guidelines suggest slightly different parameters for active surveillance candidates.

Prostate cancer is generally a slow progression disease. Don't let the "Cancer Anxiety Factor" push you into a more aggressive treatment option than is dictated by the prognosis data.

Chapter 6.
Surgery

The surgical removal of all (Radical) or part (Simple) of the prostate gland is called a **prostatectomy**. Multiple surgical approaches exist for both of these operations. A simple prostatectomy is used in the treatment of Benign Prostatic Hypertrophy, while a Radical prostatectomy is generally used in the treatment of early or intermediate stage prostate cancer. The simple prostatectomy is outside the scope of this book.

Radical prostatectomy is sometimes referred to as open prostatectomy, as the procedure sees an "opening" or incision being made in the patient's abdomen or perineal area, depending on which procedure is being undertaken: **radical retropubic prostatechtomy (RRP)** – operate via the abdomen or **radical perineal prostatectomy (RPP)** – operate via the perineal area between the scrotum and the anus.

Radical retropubic prostatectomy (RRP) is a surgical procedure in which the prostate gland is removed through a small incision in the abdomen. It is most often used to treat men who have early-stage prostate cancer. RRP is usually performed under general anaesthetic and may require blood transfusions in less than 20% of cases. Common complications of a RRP are urinary incontinence and impotence. These outcomes are dependent on the experience and skill of the surgeon, the technique used and the physical anatomy of the patient. The most common surgical approach is to make a small incision in the skin between the umbilicus and the top of the pubic bone. The important structures in the pelvic region such as the prostate, bladder, urethra, blood vessels, and nerves are identified. Nerve-sparing surgery attempts to protect the neurovascular bundles which control erections. These nerves run next to the prostate and may be damaged or destroyed during surgery, leading to impotence. An important part of the operation is to protect the cavernous nerves to minimize impotency and to maintain urinary control. During surgery, the surgeon may apply a small electrical stimulation to these nerves and measure the erectile function with a penile plethysmograph. This test aids the surgeon in identifying the nerves, which are difficult to see.

The prostate is separated from the urethra below and the bladder above, and the bladder and urethra are reconnected. The blood vessels leading to and from the prostate are then divided and tied off. The prostate, seminal vesicles, ends of the vas deferens, and, depending on oncological considerations, nerve bundles and/or pelvic lymph nodes are removed. A catheter is maintained in the urethra for up to about a week after the operation.

Radical perineal prostatectomy (RPP) has become a less popular surgical procedure due to limited access to lymph nodes and the difficulty in avoiding nerves.

Laporoscopic Radical Prostatectomy (LRP) is a modern form of radical prostatectomy which has substantially taken over from the earlier open form of surgery. A laparoscopic radical prostatectomy does not require a large incision, makes no use of retractors and does not require the abdominal wall to be parted and stretched for the duration of the operation. It is a form of "keyhole" surgery. A laparoscope is introduced into the sub-umbilical site (the area between the umbilical and pubic areas) and is used to guide the operation. The surgeon and assistant each use the other four sites (usually with up to 5mm long incisions) for the introduction of instruments. Laparoscopic radical prostatectomy and open radical prostatectomy differ only in how they access the deep pelvic area and generate operative views. In contrast to open radical prostatectomy, LPR, in the hands of a capable and experienced urological surgeon, sees very little blood loss, little post-operative pain and less chance of infection. Some LRP procedures include the use of robots. They are referred to as **Robotic-Assisted Laparoscopic Prostatectomy (RALP) or Robotic-Assisted Laparoscopic Radical Prostatectomy (RALRP)**. These are both the same procedure.

The most well-known such robot laparoscopic system is the *da Vinci*® **Prostatectomy System** (Intuitive Surgical Inc., California, USA). The manufacturer claims on their web site that 4 out of 5 prostatectomy operations in the USA are performed on their system. Over 1.5

million patients have been treated on their systems for a range of conditions. The *da Vinci*® System features a magnified 3D high-definition vision system and special wristed instruments which are able to bend and rotate far more than the human wrist. It also contains tremor filtering technology. *da Vinci*® enables the surgeon to operate with enhanced vision, precision, dexterity and control. A *da Vinci*® prostatectomy offers the following potential benefits compared to traditional laparoscopy:

More patients return to pre-surgery erectile function at 12-month checkup[13,14]

Faster return of urinary continence[14]

Lower risk of complications[1]

Less blood loss and need for a transfusion[1,8]

Less chance of nerve injury[1]

Less chance of injuring the rectum[1]

Shorter operation[8]

Less risk of deep vein thrombosis (life-threatening condition where a blood clot forms deep in the body)[1]

Shorter hospital stay[1,8]

Less chance of hospital readmission[1]

Less chance of needing follow-up surgery[1]

More details and the references listed above are accessible via Appendix 3.

An important general advantage that RALP systems offer over the open surgery technique is an improved visual access of the operative field, particularly behind the pubic bone. This is achieved by use of a laparoscope that provides bright and even illumination of the magnified field of view and an image on a monitor that is able to be viewed by the surgeon, the assistant and scrub nurses in real time. This facilitates better team work by the surgeon and his assistant and a more precise dissection, which, in turn, provides better control of potential sources of bleeding.

As is the case in open prostatectomy, robotic radical prostatectomy entails the removal of the whole prostate and seminal vesicles. They are withdrawn generally through one of the 5 mm long incisions. Occasionally, it is necessary to extend the incision to extract a larger prostate. On occasion, particularly with patients with immediate risk (advanced localised) cancer, the surgeon might remove some lymph nodes near the prostate to see if the cancer has spread beyond the prostate. If the pathologist reports cancer in the lymph nodes, the surgeon will recommend further treatment, because the cancer is no longer localised. Sampling of the lymph nodes adds further time to the length of the operation, particularly so for the RALP technique.

During the RALP procedure the patient is placed in a steep 'head down' position, which on rare occasions leads to anaesthetic complications. After the operation, the surgeon will send the tissue they removed to the laboratory. The aim of the surgery is to remove all the cancer with a safety margin of cancer free tissue around it. This safety margin is called a **clear margin**. Should the pathologist find cancerous cells at the extremity of the removed tissue or in any removed lymph node tissue, it is likely that a course of radiation will be recommended. A key consideration in deciding to undergo a RALP operation is to determine the experience of the surgeon undertaking the operation.

Surgeons, who are proficient with both keyhole systems, appear to take a similar average length of time to perform the surgery of about 150 to 180 minutes. Average blood loss in a recent study was 533ml. In a 2001 study, it was reported as being 354 +/- 250 ml. Other studies report even lower blood losses with only very few patients requiring blood transfusions. François Rozet, Jamison Jaffe, et al. reported after a comparison of conventional laparoscopic to robot assisted laparoscopic prostatectomies within their institution that the conventional technique provided comparable results to those obtained by the RALP procedure.[1]

Background of Radical Prostatectomy

Radical prostatectomy is generally regarded as the most reliable treatment to cure prostate cancer. It is considered to be the "golden standard" treatment.[2] From its introduction just after the 2nd World

War, radical prostatectomy was associated with a high percentage of patients experiencing erectile dysfunction and/or incontinence after surgery. The precise pathway of the nerves mediating erectile function was reported by Dr. Lepor in the early 80's. Based on these discoveries, Drs Walsh and Lepor described a nerve sparing radical prostatectomy which greatly improved the likelihood of preserving erectile function following surgery.[3]

Dr Lepor has been a prolific publisher of scientific studies on erectile dysfunction after a radical prostatectomy. Prior to 2000, he reported that 40% of all men undergoing the surgical procedure will develop erectile dysfunction. This was despite the fact that he co-developed the surgical procedure and has performed 4500 radical prostatectomies. He reported the likelihood that erectile function will be preserved is dependent on many criteria including age, erectile function before surgery, if both nerves can be preserved and if cardiovascular co-morbidities are present. More recently, he co-authored a paper that reported on a total of 1,110 men undergoing open radical retropubic prostatectomy by a single surgeon, found 34% were not potent, post-operatively.[4]

A 2013 paper, *'Advances in Robotic Assisted Laparoscopic Prostatectomy over Time'*, by Emma F. P. Jacobs, et al., reviewed the advances made in the perioperative management and surgical technique of RALP.[5] This is a paper which is well worth reading.

Over the years, there have been numerous subtle and substantive changes to the surgical techniques using robotic assistance or conventionally. Despite these changes in surgical technique, many men still experience erectile dysfunction and/or incontinence. The increased use of the RALP technique has seen lesser blood losses, a shorter hospital stay and has resulted in very low 6% positive margins in cases of organ confined disease. As Dr Thomas E. Ahlering, MD, of the University of California, Irvine, states on his web site, *"Prior to the Da Vinci® robot, it was very difficult to make such a clean and refined excision of the apical region of the prostate"*.[6]

An interesting table exists on the da Vinci® Surgery web site that compares patient outcomes for open, laparoscopic and da Vinci® RALP surgery. Access the web site via Appendix 3.

Outcomes and Side Effects

The 'Holy Grail' in the treatment of prostate cancer is an approach that reliably eradicates prostate cancer while preserving erectile function and urinary continence. This is an outcome that is impossible to guarantee, within the confines of present medical technology. In the main, the surgery option is only offered to men with local or advanced local disease. This increases the results for these men being cancer free years after the surgery. An Australian report [7] indicated cancer-free outcomes as follows:

After 5 years: - 75 to 85% cancer free

After 10 years: - 70 to 80% cancer free

After 15 years: - 60% cancer free

(These figures have been rounded to the nearest 5%)

Survival rates for men who have had cancer after having had surgery are also impressive:

After 5 years: - 96 to 98% survival

After 10 years: - 90 to 96% survival

After 15 years: - 81 to 82% survival

In a recently published research paper, JJ Park, et al.,[8] found that a pre-prostatectomy 3 Tesla field strength multiparametric MRI using a phased-array coil, including T2-weighted imaging (T2WI), diffusion-weighted imaging (DWI), and dynamic contrast-enhanced MRI (DCE-MRI), was a significant independent indicator of biochemical recurrence of the cancer when the results of all three techniques were combined. After a median follow-up of 26 months, biochemical recurrence developed in 22% of patients out of the 282 men in the study. This finding stresses the importance of having regular post treatment PSA testing.

Before you make a final commitment to have surgery, ask yourself the following questions:

Have you sought a second opinion?

Have you contacted a prostate cancer support group for input?

Do you fully understand the side effect risks that can significantly alter your quality of life?

Have you fully discussed your choice with your wife or partner?

Are you "blindly" following your urologist recommendation to have surgery?

Do you "just want the cancer out of my body"?

If you answered no to the first four questions and yes to the last two questions, it might be appropriate to step back and take stock of what you are facing.

Questions you should ask your surgeon after you have made a commitment to have surgery:

What exact type of surgery do you propose? (Open RRP; RPP, RLP or RALP?)

How many of these operations have you done and how many do you do a year?

What are your results? Do you keep a data base of these results?

Will you try to do the nerve sparing surgery?

Will you remove any lymph nodes?

How long does the operation take?

Should I donate my own blood prior to surgery?

When should I stop aspirin (or warfarin) prior to surgery?

What about other supplements?

How long will I be in the hospital?

How do I take care of my catheter?

When will I have my first post-operation appointment?

What if I see blood in my urine?

When do I start exercising after surgery?

What other activities can I do and when? Golf? Jogging? Bike Riding?

When can I drive? When can I return to work?

How long will I need to wear a urinary pad?

How soon will I recover an erection?

Should I use Viagra, Levitra or Cialis after surgery?

When can I have intercourse after removal of my catheter?

How long until my urinary control returns?

What fills the space of the removed prostate? Is the length of the erected penis different?

What type of ejaculation can I expect?

What is the chance of needing further treatment for cancer after surgery?

Summary – Surgery

Surgery is usually only offered to patients with prostate cancer that is confined "to the box".

Surgeons do either open or laparoscopic ("keyhole") prostatectomies with access to the prostate via the abdomen. A few surgeons have reason to access the prostate region via the perineum (between the testes and the anus).

The use of robot-assisted prostatectomies using the da Vinci® Prostatectomy is becoming more and more common.

The experience of the surgeon undertaking the procedure is a critical factor in getting a good outcome. Figures well into the hundreds of successfully procedures, in some reviews, are considered essential.

Some Factors in favour of a Prostatectomy

After active surveillance, it is concerned the most common treatment for prostate cancer that is still "confined to the box".

Keyhole surgery sees a rapid recovery and early return to work.

Pathology of the removed prostate can confirm an adequate margin, that is, no cancer cells were present on the extremity of the prostate.

It is possible to remove any cancerous tissue in nearby lymph glands or pelvic area during the procedure.

Some Factors against having a Prostatectomy

One is very dependent on the experience and skill of the surgeon.

A high percentage of patients have incontinence and impotency challenges.

Studies have shown that a biochemical recurrence of the cancer may occur in up to 22% of patients.

A possible need to harvest your blood prior to surgery.

Chapter 7.
Radiation Therapy

7.1. External Beam Radiation Therapy (EBRT)

Radiotherapy in its many forms (EBRT; IMRT; IGRT; conformal 3D-CRT; PBT; SBRT and the two formats of brachytherapy), together with radical prostatectomy remains the overwhelming treatment prescribed for the treatment of localized (early stage) and localized (intermediate risk) advanced prostate cancer. Radiotherapy is sometimes used as an adjunct therapy to other treatments, e.g. a short course of radiotherapy might follow a prostatectomy or a high dose brachytherapy procedure. Patients that present themselves with a PSA of greater than 10 and/or a Gleason score of 7 to 10, often undergo a course of hormone therapy plus EBRT, which has been shown to improve survival rates.

EBRT has been a main stream therapy for treating cancers for many decades. Its increase in use coincided with the introduction of improved linear accelerators (LINACS) in the 60's. LINACS are devices that generate the x-rays used to treat cancers. EBRT treatment protocols call for the patient's prostate to be exposed to short pulses of tightly focused beams of x-rays for a few minutes each day for five days a week for about 7 weeks. It is a painless procedure with no short term noticeable side effects.

EBRT (and its later derivatives, IMRT etc.) deliver treatment outcomes for patients with low or intermediate risk tumours, with results that are closely comparable to that of surgery or brachytherapy. EBRT has also been shown to provide long term quality of life outcomes that are again broadly similar to surgery and brachytherapy.[1,2] Patients that present with a PSA of greater than 10 and/or a Gleason score of 7 to 10, often undergo a course of hormone treatment plus EBRT, which has been shown to improve survival rates.[3]

Before the course of treatment begins, it is usual for a series of imaging procedures, such as MRI's, CT scans and normal x-rays of the pelvis/prostate area to be done, to locate the exact position, shape and size of the prostate. The radiation oncologist will calculate the exact dose to be delivered and develop a treatment plan specific to that patient. The radiation team may make a series of ink marks on the skin to assist them in directing the radiation to the prostate.

The advantages of EBRT versus surgery are:

It is less intrusive and stressful than surgery.

It avoids any risk of infection.

It is suitable for all ages and health conditions.

There is no need to harvest some of your own blood prior to undertaking surgery.

It might offer cost advantages dependent on the patient's jurisdiction.

Its disadvantage versus surgery is the need to front up each working day for about an hour for at least 7 weeks (and sometime up to 9 weeks). The patient has only a few minutes exposure to x-rays, but the set up procedures can take up to thirty minutes. For patients that are some distance from the treatment centre, the cost of travel and travel time are often not inconsequential.

EBRT generally leads to some radiation damage to the bladder and the bowel. Many EBRT patients experience mild to moderate bowel inflammation that manifests itself in the form of loose and more frequent bowel motions, and possible rectal bleeding. This might only occur six months to many years after radiation treatment concludes and may be an ongoing malady. About 3% of men develop severe and ongoing bowel problems. Rates of occurrence of incontinence and impotence are much less to those experienced by surgery patients. With EBRT, up to about half of men develop erection problems, some of which respond to remedial treatments, such as use of Viagra, etc.[4]

The skill of the radiation oncologist and the equipment used can make a marked difference in the outcomes achieved. Thus, it is important to understand _your_ radiation oncologist's success record using the same treatment parameters. With the newer variants of EBRT, outcomes are generally superior to those achieved with the older technology. This is mainly due to the ability to focus the radiation more accurately and at higher doses on the prostate and by reducing the radiation exposure to healthy adjacent tissue.

What happens in the event that the cancer growth returns in the future after initial radiation therapy?

After your initial prostate cancer treatment, the medical staff will require you to have at least 6-monthly PSA tests to monitor the reduction in your PSA level over a 12 month period to a level of somewhere between 0 and 2 ng/ml. Approximately 30% of men treated for localized prostate cancer experience a biochemical relapse after their initial treatment.[5] This suggests a need to maintain vigilance for years after initial successful treatment by regular PSA testing. Two studies after radical prostatectomies found that the BCR incidences were 32% and 15% respectively.[6,7]

If a problem exhibits itself in the form of a much higher PSA result, it is likely to be between 2 and 10 years after the original radiation treatment. (Shorter 'recurrence' periods of less than 2 years are probably 'progression' of the disease and not a recurrence). Several "salvage treatments" are available which might include radical prostatectomy, cryotherapy, high-frequency ultrasound, chemotherapy or hormone treatment. It is not possible to have further radiation therapy, due to the urethra not being able to handle the same. It is reported that a "salvage" prostatectomy is an extremely challenging procedure, with some specialists now starting to favour focused techniques like cryotherapy or HIFU (in countries were the latter technique is approved).[8]

After radiation therapy, PSA levels reach their nadir (lowest point) up to two years after treatment. A **biochemical recurrence** after radiation therapy is typically defined as three PSA increases above the nadir (lowest) PSA level measured at least two weeks apart by the same lab. A further definition, the "Phoenix consensus", calls for the nadir value plus 2 to be used for BCR. Radiation therapy is also used to treat patients with metastatic prostate cancer (cancer that has spread beyond the prostate). This relieves symptoms of bone pain, obstructions or bleeding.

Note that the definition for biochemical recurrence is different in the case of a total prostatectomy as the PSA level drops to what might be regarded as zero after the operation. A biochemical recurrence after a radical prostatectomy is regarded as being present when a PSA reading of > 0.2 ng/ml increases in each of two further tests at least two weeks apart using the same lab.[9]

We have seen that rectal damage from radiation is a real challenge for prostate cancer patients. It affects all men undergoing radiation treatment (of all types and formats) to a greater or lesser degree. There is now a product available, in many countries, that substantially eliminates the possibility of radiation damage to the bowel. At time of writing it, is not approved for use by the FDA in the USA. It's called the SpaceOAR® System – Spacing Organs At Risk. SpaceOAR® hydrogel is injected as a liquid between the prostate and rectum under ultrasound guidance. Once injected, the liquid solidifies within seconds into a hydrogel that pushes the rectum away from the prostate. The result is reduced rectal radiation during radiation therapy. The hydrogel maintains space during radiation therapy for up to three months and then liquefies, allowing it to be absorbed into and cleared from the body (within six months).

Access their web site via Appendix 3. View the graphic on SpaceOAR® on the next page.

Summary – External Beam Radiation

EBRT (and its later derivatives, IMRT etc.) deliver treatment outcomes for patients with low or intermediate risk tumours, with results that are closely comparable to that of surgery or brachytherapy.

Long term quality of life outcomes that are broadly similar to surgery and brachytherapy.

Later derivatives of EBRT generally give better outcomes than older systems.

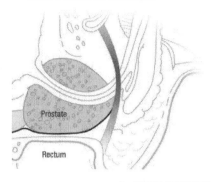 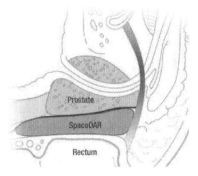

SpaceOAR Hydrogel Application
- Biocompatible
- Maintains space for ~ 3 months
- Absorbs in ~ 6 months

Image: Courtesy of Augmenix Inc.

Factors in favour of EBRT

It is less invasive than surgery with no infection risk and is likely to cost less than surgery.

It suits all ages and health conditions.

Avoids the stress of an anaesthetic and surgery.

Some Factors against EBRT

Radiation damages the urethra, et al. In cases of a recurrence of the cancer, fewer salvage treatment options are available and greater difficulties occur in undertaking these options.

The patient needs to commit to daily treatment (weekdays only) for up to ten weeks.

Possibility of rectal burning (avoidable by using the SpaceOAR® hydrogel). Also bladder difficulties such as blood in the urine, etc.

Higher risk of bladder cancer some 10 to 15 years after the radiation treatment.

7.2. 3-Dimensional Conformal Radiation Therapy, Intensity-Modulated Radiotherapy, Image-Guided Radiotherapy (3-D CRT, IMRT and IGRT) and Tomotherapy

The advance in the capabilities of imaging machines such as CT and MRI over the past two decades has led to the capability to accurately delineate tumours and adjacent normal structures in three dimensions. Improvements in radiation treatment planning software and the ability to shape the profile of the radiation beam to match that of the target by using multi-leaf collimators lead to the introduction of **3-dimensional conformal radiation therapy** and subsequently, IMRT and IGRT and more. These developments reduced the radiation to the surrounding healthy tissue and allowed a higher radiation dose to be directed at the tumour.[10]

Intensity-modulated radiation therapy (IMRT) is an advanced type of high-precision radiation that is the next generation of 3-D CRT. The LINAC (an x-ray linear accelerator) delivers precise radiation doses to malignant tumors or specific areas within the tumor under advanced computer control. The single radiation dose is delivered using a series of tiny beam –shaping devices called collimators. The collimators can be stationary or can move during treatment which allows the intensity of the radiation beam to be changed during treatment. This variance in dose intensity is called **dose modulation**, which sees different parts of the tumour and the healthy surrounding tissue, receive different radiation doses. This dose modulation provides better tumor targeting, reduced side effects, and improved treatment outcomes than the earlier 3-D CRT systems.

The pattern of radiation delivery is determined by the radiation oncologist, in conjunction with a medical physicist. They develop a treatment plan, which uses advanced computing applications to perform optimization and treatment simulation routines. The treatment plan also determines the multiple angles to be used to deliver the total radiation dose. It is advantageous to have as much energy as possible impact the tumour, whilst sparing healthy tissue by having multiple body entry points.

In IMRT, an inverse treatment plan is generally used. The inverse treatment plan sees the radiation oncologist choose the radiation doses to be delivered to different parts of the tumour and its surrounding tissue. The computer program takes the inputted data and calculates the required number of beams, their angles, etc. In traditional treatment plans, the number and angles of the beams is determined by the radiation oncologist, with the computer determining the dose level to be delivered by each of the beams.

With any cancer treatment, what is important is the outcome and to perhaps a lesser extent, the side effects that are experienced. IMRT has been in widespread use for about 10 years, after its introduction in the late 1990's. Anecdotally, it is considered vastly superior to its predecessor devices such as the EBRT and 3D confocal therapy systems. Certainly, it ensures reduced radiation exposure to healthy tissue and increased dosage to the tumour site than with earlier radiation systems. In fact, the control of the radiation beam is so good that some facilities with IMRT systems are now selectively offering IMRT as salvage treatment to men who have previously had x-ray radiation therapy.[11]

To illustrate the improvements that IMRT has provided with regard to reducing radiation damage to organs at risk, the results of a large study conducted on more than 1400 prostate cancer sufferers done at the Fox Chase Cancer Centre, Philadelphia, showed that the genitourinary side effects of the two treatments at three years post treatment were statistically similar, whereas there were lesser gastrointestinal (rectal) side effects reported for IMRT. This was despite higher doses being used for the IMRT treatments.[12] In a further study at the Fox Chase Cancer Centre, it was reported that, although 3D-CRT therapy combined with hormone therapy, produced excellent outcomes in intermediate and high risk patients, the patients treated with confocal radiation therapy were twice as likely to suffer gastrointestinal side effects compared with the group who had been treated with IMRT when measured at a mean follow up of 86 months.[13]

Image-Guided Radiation Therapy (IGRT) is a form of IMRT, which sees repeated image scans of the tumour area done by CT, MRI or PET immediately before treatment or during the treatment. The results obtained from the imaging scans are feed into the IGRT computer system for it to detect changes in the size or position of the tumour. These results are compared with the images stored in the system from the simulation done in the development of the treatment plan. The computer makes appropriate adjustments to the treatment area, thus ensuring maximum precision is made in radiation delivery.

Tomotherapy is similar to IGRT. The machine is a hybrid between a CT imaging scanner and an EBRT machine. The radiation part of the unit has the capability to rotate completely around the patient as is done by a normal CT machine. Tomo therapy machines can capture CT images of the patient's tumour immediately before treatment sessions which assists in the precision of radiation delivery. It is thought that, like standard IMRT, tomotherapy may be better at sparing healthy tissue from high radiation doses, but no clinical trials appear to have been done to compare 3D-CRT with tomotherapy in a prostate cancer setting. Tomotherapy was found to have advantages over IMRT and 3D-CRT based on the dosimetric comparison in a post-operative breast cancer study, especially in the high dose region of lung, target homogeneity and dose uniformity.[14]

Dosage

Around the world the standard dosage for radiation therapy appears to be 70.2 Gy. However, over a period of years, the dosage usually delivered in the USA has increased to 79.2 Gy, which is regarded elsewhere as dose-escalated RT. In September 2014, a trial by a group of 104 US centres, collectively known as the Radiation Therapy Oncology Group (RTOG) 0126, reported its findings. The trial compared high-dose RT (79.2 Gy) with standard-dose RT (70.2 Gy) in the treatment of more than 1500 men with intermediate-risk prostate cancer. It found that there was no significant difference in overall survival between men in the high-dose group and men in the standard-dose group (66.7% vs 65.6%). It did report higher instances in both gastrointestinal (GI) and genitourinary (GU) toxicity with the higher dose patients. However, it did report that dose escalation did improve local control and distant metastases-free and biochemical disease-free survivals, but with accompanying increased GI and GU toxicity.

Summary - 3-D CRT, IMRT and IGRT and Tomotherapy

All the above systems under the control of a good radiation oncologist provide the same or better outcomes than provided by an older EBRT system.

The use of advanced software routines, multi-leaf collimators, variations in the dose presented to different parts of the tumour, all work to minimise the radiation dose received by healthy tissue and increase the radiation dosage to the tumour site.

IGRT is able to track movements in organs whilst the patient is under treatment and adjusts the direction and intensity of the radiation dose to compensate for these movements, thus ensuring an optimal radiation session.

Increased dose delivery increases future metastases-free and biochemical disease-free survivals, but with accompanying increased GI and GU challenges.

It may be used to "top-up" the radiation dose after brachytherapy.

Some Factors in favour of 3-D CRT, IMRT and IGRT, etc.

IMRT control has now improved to the extent that it can be used in select cases of cancer recurrence in patients previously treated with radiation.

It offers less damage to healthy tissue than earlier EBRT systems. GI and GU difficulties are being lessened which supports an improved lifestyle.

Some Factors against the use of 3-D CRT, IMRT and IGRT, etc.

The patient needs to commit to daily treatment (weekdays only) for up to ten weeks.

Possibility of rectal burning (avoidable by using the SpaceOAR® hydrogel). Also possible bladder difficulties such as blood in the urine, etc. as a result of radiation 'scatter'.

A lower risk of bladder cancer when compared with older EBRT systems years after the radiation treatment.

7.3. Stereotactic Body Radiotherapy (SBRT)

Stereotactic radiation is a specialised form of external beam radiation therapy (EBRT). It uses focused radiation beams to target the tumour. The radiation dose is delivered with extreme accuracy by utilising detailed imaging, computerised 3-D treatment planning and precise treatment set up. It is a treatment for low and intermediate risk prostate cancer patients. There are two types of stereotactic radiation: Stereotactic radiosurgery (SRS): a single or multiple stereotactic radiation treatments of the brain or spine. SRS is outside the scope of this book. **Stereotactic body radiation therapy (SBRT):** one or several stereotactic radiation treatments to parts of the body, excluding the brain or spine.

A number of machines are available for SBRT treatment of the prostate. These include the Rapid Arc (marketed as a volumetric arc therapy system); the **CyberKnife**®; Elektra Synergy®; Tomo Therapy; Varian Trilogy® the Siemens Oncor® and Artiste® and the Novalis X-Knife® Tx radiation system. All these systems use x-rays (photons) to irradiate the tumour. Most of these systems also incorporate the capability to move the radiation dose being delivered to conform to movements of the tumour due to organ movement, e.g. rectal or bladder. The image guidance systems identify the exact position in the prostate of three implanted gold seed markers called **fiducials**. (These are implanted in a process similar to biopsy sampling). The fiducial positions are continually reported by the image guidance system to the intensity modulated beam system that is shaped to fit and surround the prostate gland, aiming at the prostate gland continuously as the gantry rotates through 360 degrees around the patient. One such specialised beam system is called **RapidArc**®.[15] This system, when combined with the Novalis Tx, contains a treatment planning algorithm that simultaneously changes three parameters during treatment:

Rotation speed of the gantry.

Shape of the treatment aperture using the movement of multi-leaf collimator leaves.

Delivery dose rate.

The RapidArc® volumetric modulated arc therapy system differs from other systems like helical IMRT or intensity-modulated arc therapy (IMAT) as it delivers its dose to the whole volume of the tumour (and it safety margin) rather than slice by slice as in other systems. The accuracy of these new technologies allows the margin around the prostate to be reduced, thus significantly reducing the side effects to the rectum and bladder.

The American Society for Therapeutic Radiology and Oncology (ASTRO) Emerging Technology Committee's report on SBRT for prostate cancer is recommended reading for the technically-minded.[16] The key advantage of SBRT is it delivers the right amount of radiation to the cancer in a shorter amount of time (usually 5 treatment sessions of about 15 minutes each as an outpatient) and generally more accurately than other radiation treatments.[17] Dr Chris King of UCLA was an early pioneer in the use of SBRT and in 2010 published an update of his clinical SBRT trial, now with 2.7 years median follow-up, where he has shown that the late side effects are minimal, similar in nature to those described for standard external beam radiotherapy, and often less frequent than seen with the standard radiotherapy courses.[18]

With prostate cancer, the proximity of the bowel and bladder might limit the radiation dose applied. Radiation exposure to the rectum and bladder is considered equal or better than brachytherapy and cancer control outcomes are reported as equivalent to those of brachytherapy, conventional external beam radiation or surgery. The side effects experienced are generally somewhat greater than those experienced with conventional external beam radiotherapy. The cost of the procedure was found to be significantly lower than IMRT.[19] (This study covers the period 2008 to 2011, when SBRT was in its initial years of use. It is likely that outcomes have improved with better operator experience and training since 2011).

The CyberKnife® Robotic Radiosurgery System delivers radiotherapy to the patient with greater precision and accuracy than standard radiotherapy systems. It consists of a small linear particle accelerator that produces the radiation beam and a robotic arm which allows the energy to be targeted and delivered to any part of the body from any direction. The mounting of the radiation source on the robot arm allows maximum freedom to rapidly move the source to deliver radiation doses to the patient from multiple directions sequentially. It also includes an image guidance system allowing the system to compensate for minor organ movement. The system incorporates x-ray imaging cameras which are mounted on supports around the patient allowing real time x-ray images to be obtained.

The CyberKnife® has been around for nearly 25 years with more recent models being vastly superior to the earlier models. The first system was installed in Perth in West Australia in 2013 and offers prostate cancer treatment for Australian and a limited number of international patients.[20] Although its name may suggest surgery, the CyberKnife® does not involve cutting at all. It is purely a radiation delivery device, albeit a very sophisticated one. The CyberKnife® has treated more than 100,000 cancer patients with more than 5,000 having been treated for prostate cancer.

What questions should I ask my Specialist about external beam radiation therapy (all variants)?

Will I be radioactive?

Will I be treated as an outpatient? (No hospital stay)

How many radiation sessions will I need?

What can I do to prepare myself for the radiation treatment?

What can I do to speed my recovery?

Should I get a second opinion? If not, why not?

Is the radiation painful and are their short term side-effects?

How can I avoid radiation damage to the rectum?

What are the health risks from radiation? Erectile dysfunction? Incontinence? Rectal damage?

What form of machine (EBRT; 3-D Conformal; IMRT; etc.) might be used for my radiation? Is it the best available to me? If not, why not?

If there is a future recurrence of the cancer, what 'salvage' treatments are available?

Is there a prostate cancer support group that you might recommend?

Am I likely to get as good an outcome as: surgery; brachytherapy (both types), other treatments?

What will the radiation sessions cost? What percentage will be covered by Medicare? What percentage will be covered by my private health insurance? What percentage will I have to bear out of my own pocket?

What if I have had previous prostate surgery, TURP or bladder neck incision?

Will I still be able to father children after the radiation session?

After the radiation treatment is complete, what is the follow up procedure? Short term? Longer term?

Summary – SBRT

Radiation exposure to the rectum and bladder is considered equal or better than brachytherapy and cancer control outcomes are reported as equivalent to those of brachytherapy, conventional external beam radiation or surgery. The side effects experienced are generally somewhat greater than those experienced with conventional external beam radiotherapy.

A key attribute of the use of SBRT systems in treating prostate cancer is the escalation of dose which allows a full dosage to be delivered in 5 or less radiation sessions. The sophisticated control of the radiation beam that is usually delivered through 360° with the ability of the system to compensate for organ movement during radiation delivery, provides acceptable radiation exposure to the prostate.

Some Factors in Favour of SBRT

The benefit of only needing up to five radiation sessions.

The cost is likely to be much lower than IMRT and other x-ray radiation systems.

Some Factors against the use of SBRT

The jury is still out as to the long term GI and GU impact of SBRT.

7.4. Proton Beam Therapy

A Brief Look at Standard Radiation Therapy

Everyone has had an x-ray at some time or other. These days CT scans are done as a diagnostic aid on a regular basis. These all involve parts of the body being irradiated with x-rays in the form of photons. A normal chest x-ray provides the patient with about the same radiation dose as would be received in 10 days from background radiation. A CT scan would provide many times this level of radiation. Radiation therapy for treating cancer provides considerably higher radiation exposure to the patient than via a CT scan, with the energy in the radiation beam irradiating healthy as well as cancerous tissue before and after the tumour. This leads to undesirable side effects and in worst cases, triggers secondary cancers due to the exposure of the healthy cells to high doses of radiation.

All radiation therapy works by damaging the DNA of the cells that the radiation interacts with, and the goal is to deposit as much energy (or dose) as possible to the tumour site while minimizing the dose and associated damage to the surrounding healthy tissues. Many approaches have been taken to reduce the radiation damage to healthy tissue adjacent to the tumour. These include irradiating the tumour from different angles; modification of the beam to match the tumour shape; and modulating the intensity of the radiation delivered to different parts of the tumour. More recently, technical advances have allowed the tumour to be irradiated from all around the patient. Even with these advances in radiation delivery, the collateral damage to healthy tissue and the limitations on the maximum dose exposure to healthy tissue are still a concern.

What is Proton Therapy?

Proton therapy is an external-beam radiation therapy technique not dissimilar to conventional high energy x-rays. The difference is that protons are heavy charged particles that deposit their radiation dose in a very precise targeted manner. When protons enter the body, they have little lateral scatter in the body tissue with the beam hardly broadening. They leave a minimal amount of energy along their path as they pass through healthy tissue on their way to the target tumour. When they reach the target depth (the tumour), the protons deposit a large focused amount of energy on the target and then dissipate, leaving almost no energy beyond the targeted depth. The protons, which are relatively high mass charged particles, damage the DNA of cells, ultimately causing their death or interfering with their ability to proliferate. Cancerous cells are particularly vulnerable to attacks on DNA because of their high rate of division and their reduced abilities to repair DNA damage due to their poor blood supply, etc.

This ability of the protons to deposit almost all of their energy at a specific depth is referred to as the Bragg Peak Effect which was discovered by William Bragg in 1904. In modern proton therapy systems, the depth of the Bragg Peak is accurately controlled by changing the energy of the protons, thus allowing clinicians to precisely tailor the proton dose to the specific depth and shape of the tumour while minimizing the dose to surrounding healthy tissue. The advantages of proton therapy over conventional radiotherapy are significant in areas of the body with critical adjacent structures such as the eye, brain, base of the skull, spine, and prostate. These advantages also extend to paediatric cancer patients.

Protons of different energies with Bragg peaks at different depths are usually applied to treat the entire tumour.

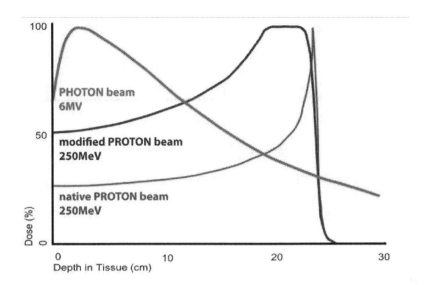

Image: Courtesy of Wikipedia

In a typical treatment plan for proton therapy, the Spread Out Bragg Peak (SOBP, dashed blue line - see the image on the next page), is the therapeutic radiation distribution. The SOBP is the sum of several individual Bragg peaks (thin blue lines) at staggered depths. The depth-dose plot of an x-ray beam of photons (red line) is provided for comparison. The pink area represents the additional dose delivered by x-ray radiotherapy which can be the source of damage to normal tissues and of secondary cancers, particularly of the skin.

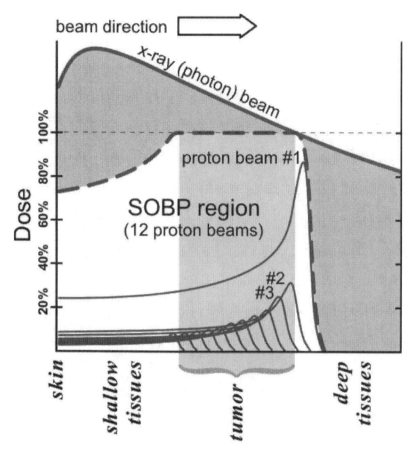

Image: Courtesy of Wikipedia

So How Does it Work?

Protons are positively charged particles – the nucleus of the hydrogen atom. Free protons are produced by ionisation of hydrogen atoms into positively charged protons and negatively charged electrons stripped from a hydrogen gas supply. The protons are injected via a vacuum tube into a linear accelerator, and in a few microseconds, their energy reaches 7 million electron volts. Free protons enter the centre of the synchrotron or cyclotron, and are guided in a circular path by a powerful magnet and are accelerated to higher and higher energies. As they gain energy they spiral outwards to the edge of the cyclotron magnet by which time their energy has increased to a total of 70 million to 250 million electron volts, which is sufficient to reach any part of the patient's body. When they achieve speeds of about two-thirds of the speed of light (100,000 miles per second), a high voltage deflects them out of the system into a beam line, which via a vacuum line guided by other magnets, presents the proton beam to the treatment room. Prostate cancer patients are treated in a gantry treatment room with the gantry rotatable through 360 degrees, which allows the beam to be delivered at any angle. The whole system is controlled by a network of computers and extensive safety systems and protocols. The protons finally enter the nozzle system where the beam is shaped as it passes through a patient specific aperture, before it reaches a compensator that exactly reflects the shape and size of one half of the patient's prostate. Passage through the compensator shapes the protons into a precise and unique 3-D profile with delivery of the most effective radiation dose in that profile to the prostate. The cell damage inflicted by the proton radiation is maximized within the tumour itself, by adjusting the energy of the protons during the treatment.

Most proton therapy systems include a patient position verification system that is interfaced to a treatment planning system (or an oncology information system). This facilitates the integration of the treatment plan with the reconstructed radiographs that enable patient positioning to within sub-millimetre accuracy.

A Short History of Proton Beam Therapy

Dr Robert Wilson first proposed the use of protons for cancer treatment in 1946 when he was working on the design of the Harvard Cyclotron Laboratory (HCL). In 1951, the first clinical treatments were performed at the Berkeley Radiation Laboratory in the USA using linear accelerators, which were designed for physics research and the space program. Ten years later collaboration began between HCL and the Massachusetts General Hospital (MGH) to pursue proton therapy. Over the next 40 years, this program progressed proton beam therapy while treating almost 10,000 patients before the Cyclotron was replaced by a new system at MGH in 2002. In 1990, the first clinical system able to address a wide range of cancers was commissioned at the Loma Linda University Medical Centre (LLUMC) in Loma Linda, California. However, the cost, size, and complexity of proton therapy systems greatly limited their widespread clinical use. By 2010 these facilities were joined by an additional seven regional hospital-based proton therapy centres in the United States, and many more worldwide. The number of these centres is rapidly growing with about 31 presently treating patients for prostate cancer and another 10 likely to start treating patients during 2014 and 2015. At least another dozen centres are in the advanced planning stage. See Appendix 5 for a comprehensive list of worldwide Proton Therapy Centres together with their contact details. A number of additional centres exist that only have a fixed beam system used exclusively for ocular, and other head cancers. This escalation in the demand for proton beam treatment facilities has been fired by the ability of the technology to treat patients with otherwise untreatable cancers (brain stem, etc.); for treatments that limit potentially serious treatment side effects (secondary cancer formation, etc.) and improved lifestyle outcomes.

The use of PBT is due to accelerate even further following commencement of the installation of the next generation of systems that are far cheaper to buy, install and run; requiring far less physical space and radiation shielding. They also incorporate additional technological capabilities over some earlier systems. The cost of these new 'compact' systems is typically in the order of US$40 - $80 million versus US$150 - $250 million for the larger systems, which are truly huge in size. Gantries require a three-story building in which to house them, with two stories typically below ground level to offer increased radiation shielding.

Latest Developments in Proton Therapy

The Holy Grail for the radiation oncologist is the ability to deliver the maximum dose of radiation to the malignant tumour, while limiting damage to healthy surrounding tissue. Easily expressed, but it is very challenging to deliver in practice. Proton beam therapy gets very close to meeting this goal. A successful research project at a leading physics research institute in Switzerland, almost 10 years ago, made a giant step towards reaching the Holy Grail, when they announced a new procedure called the Spot-Scanning technique. This dynamic, 3-D conforming radiation therapy procedure made it possible for a higher radiation dose to be applied to a tumour, with reduced damage to the surrounding healthy tissue for most of the irradiated tumours. This technique is now more generally known as **Pencil Beam Scanning (PBS)**. It allows a charged-particle beam, with particular properties (intensity, size, position, etc.) to be positioned very precisely at any desired spot within a tumour for a specified time and energy level. The technique allows numerous spots to be irradiated. Each spot is individually monitored to ensure the desired radiation dose is applied uniformly within the tumour. This extremely precise and homogeneous irradiation provides outstanding results, considering the generally irregular shape of tumours. Pencil Beam Scanning is likely to be a feature in all new systems being installed worldwide.

To date only a few facilities have PBS capability to treat prostate cancer, including the MD Anderson Proton Therapy Centre in Texas. Their complex treatment planning systems and an intricate set of magnets focus a narrow proton beam and essentially "paint" a radiation dose layer by layer. This leaves healthy tissue and other adjacent critical areas of the body unharmed. This Centre also pioneered the introduction of intensity modulated proton therapy (IMPT) which they use to treat complex or concave tumours adjacent to the spinal cord or head and throat locations.

The availability of the new generation of 'compact' proton beam systems sees them being installed by private radiation groups. They are also placed in facilities with little space or access to the huge capital sums needed to install multi-gantry systems. This can only put downward pressure on the costs of undertaking proton therapy. Another outcome is that this therapy is becoming more "mainstream" with the result that an increasing number of health insurers are likely to cover the cost of this form of cancer treatment as the costs decline. The escalation in the number of cancer treatment centres, which have proton beam therapy systems, will put a stop to the view that proton therapy is an experimental treatment and allow this treatment modality to become a truly "mainstream" treatment in the eyes of all.

What radiation dose might be needed?

Radiation oncologists refer to nominal radiation and effective biological doses which are both measured in Gray (Gy). The biological effective dose also takes into account how the dose was deposited. A typical therapy dose for the destruction of a tumour is approximately 60 to 78 Gy.

Dr Cho, who was responsible for my treatment at the National Cancer Centre, Seoul, South Korea replied to my post-treatment query regarding the dosage I had received, confirming that the biological effective dose is all important. He went on to say:

"You have definitely received a less nominal total dose of 7000 cGy delivered in 28 fractions over 5.5 weeks instead of 7800 cGy in 39 fractions over 8 weeks. However, the biological effective doses (which are more important than the nominal doses) are about the same between these two dose levels. If 7800 cGy are delivered within 5.5 weeks (279 cGy x 28 fractions) instead of 8 weeks, it will be too toxic to tolerate. Considering the recovery mechanism of the human body, we have to adjust the total dose depending on overall treatment time, 5.5 weeks vs. 8 weeks. In summary, 7000 cGy/28 fractions/5.5 weeks are equivalent to 7800 cGy/39 fractions/8 weeks in terms of biological effectiveness".

By way of background, I opted for the 28 fraction treatment rather than their standard treatment of 39 fractions usually offered to international prostate cancer patients, due to a time constraint I had back in Australia. Interestingly, most Korean prostate cancer patients undergo the 28 fraction regime.

Why choose proton therapy?

Undoubtedly, the chief advantage of proton beam therapy over other radiation treatments for prostate cancer lies in its ability to direct high energy radiation to the tumour alone, whilst minimising the exposure of healthy tissue to this potentially damaging high radiation dose. This minimizes the risk of impotence, and incontinence and also lessons the risk and severity of rectal burning/bleeding.

What does the literature tell us?

It has been shown that higher doses of radiation therapy provide better outcomes in extending the percentage of patients who remain recurrence free of prostate cancer.[21,22] It is generally considered that proton beam treatment, in which high doses of radiation can be focussed specifically on the tumour, yield good outcomes.[23] Its ability to escalate the dose, in some instances, has been shown to achieve a higher probability of "cure" than conventional radiotherapy. These include ocular tumours, skull base and spinal column tumours and inoperable sarcomas.[24]

There is another class of treatment (which includes paediatric and prostate cancers) where the increased precision of proton therapy is used to reduce unwanted side effects, by limiting the dose to normal tissue. In these cases, patients are prescribed similar proton radiation doses to those used in conventional radiation therapy, with similar clinical outcomes being achieved. There is convincing clinical data that demonstrate the advantage of sparing developing organs in children by using protons. This minimizes the exposure of healthy tissue to radiation, and results in less long term damage to the child. Conventional radiotherapy can effect normal growth in children with cancer.[25]

A historical review of actual patients treated with proton beam therapy or x-rays at Harvard to judge the risk of secondary malignancies from the radiation treatment was concluded in 2008. The study authors reported that there was a 50% lower risk of developing a secondary malignancy among patients treated with PBT versus x-rays.[26] A further study found that proton therapy reduced the risk of a secondary cancer by 26% to 39% compared to IMRT.[27]

In 2007, a Proton Task Force of the American Society of Radiation Oncology (ASTRO) was assembled to evaluate PBT. This body reported its findings in April 2012 after reviewing all pertinent data up until November 2009. It reviewed a host of cancer types treated by PBT including prostate cancer. It concluded *"Current data do not provide sufficient evidence to recommend PBT in lung cancer, head and neck cancer, GI malignancies (which includes prostate cancer), and paediatric non-CNS malignancies"*. It further concluded that *"In paediatric CNS malignancies PBT appears superior to photon approaches, but more data is needed."*[28]

There are a number of studies that suggest that the apparent small benefits of PBT might be the result of inconsistent patient set-up and internal organ movement during treatment. These two circumstances may offset the PBT advantage of increased precision. (My experience at the National Cancer Centre in Seoul suggests that patient set up was very precise. Some ten minutes were taken to set the beam entry position (via each hip) using x-ray evaluation in two planes (above and from the side) with these images superimposed on a stored CT scan image. This protocol ensured that for each treatment, I was physically in exactly the same position to within millimetre accuracy. I also had to endure the placement of a condom covered probe up the rectum before each treatment, with this 'device' inflated with water to press the prostate forward into a reproducible position each day. This 10 second procedure was a little challenging the first time I underwent it, but became much less so, (except for the one occasion when a new therapist under training did his first live insertion of the device).

The 'The Wall Street Journal' of 13 December 2013, reported the findings of a study published in the Journal of the National Cancer Institute that proton-beam therapy provided no long-term benefit over traditional radiation despite far higher costs. The data for the study came from an analysis of 30,000 Medicare (USA) beneficiaries. These findings have added to the heated debate among urologists, radiation oncologists and health-care administrators as to the cost to benefit of proton beam therapy versus standard radiation therapies or surgery. The main debate has been over ongoing side effects of the various treatment modalities.

Several major US proton centres, led by the Massachusetts General Hospital and University of Pennsylvania, in 2012 launched a phase 3 randomized trial of IMRT vs PBT for localized low and low-intermediate risk prostate cancer, with the following primary outcome to be measured at 24 months following radiation:

Efficacy of PBT vs. IMRT

Compare the reduction in mean EPIC bowel scores for men with low or low-intermediate risk prostate cancer treated with PBT versus IMRT (where higher scores represent better outcomes).

The secondary outcomes to be measured at 24 months after radiation was concluded are:

Disease Specific Quality of Life (Assess the effectiveness of PBT versus IMRT for men with low or low-intermediate risk prostate cancer in terms of disease-specific quality of life as measured by patient-reported outcomes, perceptions of care and adverse events).

Cost Effectiveness of PBT versus IMRT (Assess the cost-effectiveness of PBT versus IMRT under current conditions and model future cost-effectiveness for alternative treatment delivery and cost scenarios).

Radiation Dose and Bowel, Urinary and Erectile Function (Develop predictive models to examine the associations between selected metrics of individual radiation dose distributions and patient reported bowel, urinary and erectile function).

Identification and Evaluation Biomarkers of prostate cancer behaviour (Identify and evaluate biomarkers of prostate cancer behaviour and response to radiotherapy).

Long Term Survival (Assess longer-term – 10 year) rates of disease-specific and overall survival as well as development of lasting effects such as second cancers.

The study will report in 2016 and its findings are eagerly awaited by the medical profession. What it will not report on are the outcomes of patients receiving PBT treatment using pencil beam scanning and other PBT innovations provided by the newer "second-generation" PBT, which have only recently been introduced.

A paper titled *"Proton beam therapy and localized prostate cancer: current status and controversies"* by J A Efstathiou et al., reviews the position of proton beam versus other radiographic treatments very thoroughly.[29] You can access it via Appendix 3 later in the book. Another interesting statistic is the extent to which PBT centres allocate their treatment slots to prostate cancer versus other conditions. A 2004 analysis concluded that 26% of treatments at proton beam centres worldwide were for prostate cancer. Some individual centres have reported their prostate cancer time slots to be around half of those available or slightly higher.

The dose/volume graph, that follows, demonstrates the dose to the rectum with prostate radiation; the red colour illustrates the excess radiation dose deposited in the rectal wall with x-rays versus PBT; (35% less dose to the bladder, 59% less dose to the rectum).[30]

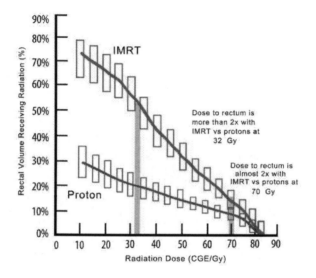

Radiation Dose to the Rectum: PBT vs. x-ray

Image: Courtesy of the University of Florida

Use of the hydrogel SpaceOAR® (referred to earlier in the book) would substantially reduce the possibility of rectal damage by any proton or photon-based radiation treatment. This product is still not available in many countries, but as its availability increases, it will become a regular addition to many radiation treatment protocols.

What possible questions should I ask my Specialist about proton beam radiation therapy?

(In some countries there are no or few PBT treatment centres. Thus, it is highly likely that many doctors and specialists (urologists, oncologists or radiologists included) will not be fully or even partially familiar with proton beam radiation, so bear this in mind when you review the possible questions below. Some questions might be appropriate and others might not be at all relevant dependant on the knowledge and experience of the doctor as far as PBT is concerned).

Are you familiar with the technique of PBT?

Do you have any experience as regards PBT? If yes, how many of your patients have had PBT? What were their outcomes? Were the outcomes better than IMRT, worse than IMRT or were they about the same?

What short term side effects did they experience?

What longer term side effects did they experience as regards erectile dysfunction, incontinence and rectal bleeding? Are there any other lasting side effects?

Were any of these patients treated on a PBT system that included Pencil Beam Scanning?

If so, were their outcomes different to those treated by IMRT? By other PBT systems?

How many radiation sessions will I need?

What can I do to prepare myself for the radiation treatment?

What can I do to speed my recovery?

If you don't recommend PBT or have no specialised knowledge of the technique, is there someone you could recommend me to? Are they local? Are they overseas?

Should I get a second opinion about possible PBT? If not, why not?

Do you use or recommend SpaceOAR® hydrogel so as to lessen or avoid radiation damage to the rectum?

If there is a future recurrence of the cancer, what 'salvage' treatments are available?

Is there a prostate cancer support group that you might recommend?

Am I likely to get as good an outcome as: surgery; brachytherapy (both types), other treatments?

What will the radiation sessions cost? What percentage will be covered by Medicare? What percentage will be covered by my private health insurance? What percentage will I have to bear out of my own pocket?

What if I have had previous prostate surgery, TURP or bladder neck incision?

Will I still be able to father children after the radiation session?

After the radiation treatment is complete, what is the follow up procedure? Short term? Longer term?

Summary – Proton Beam Therapy

Proton therapy is an external-beam radiation therapy technique not dissimilar to conventional high energy x-rays used in EBRT and IMRT systems. The difference is that protons are heavy charged particles that deposit their radiation dose in a very precise targeted manner. When protons enter the body, they have little lateral scatter in the body tissue with the beam hardly broadening.

The effectiveness of proton therapy is found in the ability of the protons to deposit almost all of their energy at a specific depth (the Bragg Peak Effect). Precisely within the tumour (or overall prostate), not before or after it, as is the case with the x-ray radiation methods.

Pencil beam scanning allows very precise delivery of the energy of the proton beam, to very small targets with the energy being released at specific depths. A single treatment might see the required dosage delivered uniformly to the target area and depth by a large number of overlapping 'sub-beams'.

Some Factors in favour of PBT

Radiation exposure to the bladder and rectum were found in a University of Florida study to be 35% and 59% lower respectively, for PBT versus IMRT.

Less healthy tissue is impacted by PBT.

Systems with pencil beam scanning capability provide further improved control and delivery of the energy beam to the target than "standard" PBT systems.

Generally less risk of impotence and incontinence compared to other radiation treatments.

Some Factors against PBT

The high cost of treatment is prohibitive to most people who don't have the treatment cost substantially or fully covered by a health fund.

With relatively few PBT facilities around the world, the patient might be away from home for 7 to 11 weeks and incur significant accommodation and travel costs.

Like all forms of radiation treatment, salvage procedures are compromised somewhat, should there be a recurrence of the cancer in future years.

7.5. Low Dose Rate Brachytherapy (Seeds)

Brachytherapy is a form of prostate cancer treatment in which ionizing radiation is delivered via radioactive material placed a short distance from, or within, the tumour. The unusual name for the procedure is derived from the Greek word *brachys* which means brief or short. There are two formats of brachytherapy. One (low dose rate brachytherapy) involves the ultrasound and template-guided insertion of radioactive seeds into the gland. The other (high dose rate brachytherapy) involves the short term insertion of radioactive needles or rods into the prostate gland with a repeat treatment generally done within 12 hours.

Seed brachytherapy partially went out of vogue 20 or 30 years ago, mainly due to the imprecise placement of the radioactive seeds into the prostate, clinician radiation exposure, etc. Other reasons were the improved performance of external radiation beam treatment (EBRT) and improvements in nerve-sparing technique in prostatectomy. The early 1990's saw introduction of improved transrectal ultrasonography (TRUS) together with the development of a guidance template that led to the introduction of percutaneous brachytherapy for the treatment of localized prostate cancer. This technique offered a significant advantage over EBRT in allowing higher radiation doses to the prostate with the benefit of reduced recurrence of prostate cancer over time.

The seeds that are implanted are about the size of a grain of rice with the number being implanted being dependant on the size of the prostate gland (and other factors). Typically 60 to 120 seeds are permanently inserted in the prostate. These seeds are inserted through the skin between the scrotum and the anus using 20 or more needles via a template. Before the procedure, the specialist will plan the positioning of the seeds in the prostate to ensure all cancerous areas are in immediate proximity to the radioactive seeds. The procedure is generally done under general anaesthetic and requires an overnight stay in hospital.

Patients undergoing LDR brachytherapy should have a prostate size of less than 60 cc (ml). If the prostate is larger, it is possible that areas of the gland are shielded by the pelvic bones, thus reducing the effectiveness of the radiation. In some instances, patients with prostate volumes of greater than 60cc, undergo hormone therapy for three months to reduce the size of the prostate to a size more suited to LDR brachytherapy. Patients with strong evidence (from biopsy results) that the cancer is fully contained within the prostate and meet low risk criteria (stage T1-T2a cancer; PSA 10 ng/ml or less and a Gleason score of 6 or less) are treated with brachytherapy alone (monotherapy). Typical prescription doses for monotherapy are 145 Gray for iodine (I)$^{-125}$ and 120-125 Gray for palladium (Pd)$^{-103}$.

Brachytherapy candidates where there is a high risk that the cancer has migrated from the prostate or who have at least two of the following criteria (stage higher than T2a cancer; PSA greater than 10 ng/ml and a Gleason score of 7 or higher) should undergo supplementary radiation by IMRT. Many urologists err on the side of conservatism, by recommending intermediate risk candidates to also undergo supplementary radiation.

Cancer cells grow by dividing much more quickly than normal cells. This rapid increase in cancer cells makes them most susceptible to the effects of radiation. Therefore the radiation released from the brachytherapy seeds will kill the rapidly dividing cancer cells. Healthy cells will be less affected by the radiation emitted by the seeds.

The isotopes most commonly used for permanent implanted seeds are iridium (Ir)$^{-192}$, iodine (I)$^{-125}$ and palladium (Pd)$^{-103}$, which have half-lives of 74, 59 and 17 days respectively. It is thus important that the patient should not hold babies or young children on their laps for three to four months after the seeds have been inserted, because of the radiation exposure to children. Similarly, close proximity to pregnant women should also be minimised. Iridium (Ir)$^{-192}$ delivers higher dosages of radiation than the other radio isotopes noted above. All three isotope seeds lose all their effective radiation within less than nine months after insertion.

The advantages of low dose brachytherapy are:

It's a minimally invasive one-off procedure.

It offers lower risk of impotence, urinary incontinence and bowel problems.

Patients are usually able to return to their normal activities within a few days.

The disadvantages are:

A need to screen your urine for two weeks after the procedure, to "capture" any seeds that may migrate into the urethra.

The possibility of the seeds migrating to elsewhere in the body, e.g. the lungs.

Possibility of a need to have a urinary catheter in place for up to a few weeks after the procedure (In as many as a reported 15% of cases).

Urinary urgency and increased frequency.

Potential impact on social and family interactions as mentioned above.

Other side effects are:

Short Term

Bruising and soreness between the legs where the needles have entered the body.

Blood in urine and semen.

A feeling of constipation due to swelling of the prostate or conversely, a feeling of a need to open one's bowels.

All these generally pass after a few weeks.

Longer Term

Some rectal bleeding occurs due to inflammation of the rectum (proctitis) in about 2% of patients.

Narrowing of the urethra sometimes occurs, somewhat restricting urinary flow.

(An excellent web site on LDR brachytherapy is accessible via Appendix 3).

The Prostate Cancer Results Study Group (P. Grimm, et al.) was formed in the USA three years ago to review 18,000 papers published over the period 2000 to 2010 in order to undertake a statistical comparative analysis of PSA free survival outcomes for patients with low, intermediate and high risk prostate cancer treatment by EBRT, brachytherapy and/or ADT. Their results suggested that brachytherapy provides superior outcomes in terms of biochemical-free progression for low risk patients. In intermediate risk patients, the combination of EBRT and brachytherapy appeared to be equivalent to brachytherapy alone, whereas in high-risk patients, a combination of EBRT, brachytherapy, with or without ADT, appeared to give better outcomes than mono-treatment protocols.[31]

Two advantages of seed brachytherapy are the greater sparing of the rectum brought about by the rapid reduction in the radiation dose delivered and the ability to provided higher initial dosage when compared to photon radiation techniques such as EBRT or IMRT. A further advantage is that in the years following the LDR brachytherapy as a monotherapy procedure, it is possible to have surgery or other salvage treatments.

LDR brachytherapy is performed as a two stage technique or in real time using loose seeds. The two-stage technique, (often referred to as the "Seattle Technique" after Grimm and Blasko from Seattle, who pioneered the technique in the late 1980s), is the most common technique used in the USA, the UK and many other countries. It requires two clinic visits and anaesthetic; the first being a pre-planning visit, with the second visit being for the actual implant procedure. It provides excellent disease free survival data at 12 years, with outcomes comparable to surgery. In about 2000, Louis Potters, of the New York Prostate Institute, developed his single visit intraoperative dynamic approach whilst working at Memorial Sloane Kettering Cancer Centre. This technique, known as the "Potters' Approach", is also able to treat larger prostates (due to less pubic arch interference). The Potters' Approach provides better control and flexibility for seed placement to that previously available. It also provides better dosimetry outcomes as well as minimising radiation exposure to the urethra and the rectum. Patients have minimal discomfort and a rapid return to normal activity. This highlights the benefits provided by LDR brachytherapy when compared with more "radical" treatments.

In January 2012, an article by Stephen E. M. Langley and Robert W. Laing was published which outlined a new real-time prostate brachytherapy technique using stranded and loose seeds.[32] Use of the 4D Brachytherapy protocol (as it is called) sees a combination of stranded seeds inserted around the periphery of the prostate gland and loose seeds placed within the centre of the prostate in a single stage real time process. A standard ultrasound scan, together with a web-based nomogram allows the number of stranded and loose seeds required for the procedure, to be determined. The procedure, performed by two clinicians working together, is usually completed in less than 45 minutes (compared with 60 to 120 minutes for a two-stage procedure). It provides better dosimetry and clinical outcomes with lesser side effects in comparison with the more common two stage protocols used.

The use of stranded seeds (in most LDR brachytherapy procedures) reduces the risk of their migration from the prostate gland to elsewhere in the body. The placement of loose seeds in the centre of the prostate gland optimises the radioactive dose to cancerous areas of the prostate whilst minimising the radiation to tissue surrounding the prostate. Stranded seeds are woven into a strand of absorbable material to help maintain their position. It is likely that x-rays will be taken during the implant procedure to check on their precise position of the inserted seeds. A CT scan is also likely after the procedure has been completed. In most instances, the patient is provided with a course of medication to be taken for a period after the procedure. These might include an alpha blocker such as Tamsulosin (Flomax®) which helps to relax the swollen muscles of the prostate, reduces pressure on the urethra and improves urinary flow. Additionally, an anti-inflammatory painkiller may be prescribed that again reduces inflammation and pain. An antibiotic is usually also taken to minimise the chances of infection. After the procedure it is likely that the patient will have some urinary retention in the form of an almost constant desire to urinate and an inability to do so. This in turn causes abdominal discomfort. Most clinics teach the patient to catheterise themselves using sterile disposable catheters, thus avoiding return visits to the clinic or their GP. Within a few weeks the urination difficulty is like to reduce and the need for catheterisation will pass.

Research suggests that erectile dysfunction will occur in about 20% of patients undergoing LDR brachytherapy. It is reported that about 80% of these cases respond very well to Viagra or similar medication. About 10% of patients experience minor bowel problems such as urgency and/or diarrhoea. These usually dissipate within a month or so of the insertion of the seeds.

What is PSA Bounce?

PSA levels decline to about 0.5 ng/ml over a period of some months after a successful seed implant, with some variability from patient to patient. Some patients, after the initial fall in PSA value, experience a rise in their PSA some 1 to 2 years after a successful seed implant. This increase is seen in up to 30% of cases with the increase in PSA value usually being in the 0.5 – 1.5 ng/ml range. In rare cases, it may rise to higher than 10 ng/ml. This phenomenon is referred to as PSA Bounce and is not preventable. Its occurrence does not suggest a poorer outcome from the seed implant procedure. The reason for a PSA Bounce occurring does not appear to be fully understood.

What Questions should I ask my Specialist about LDR Brachytherapy?

Could my prostate be too big to do a seed implant?

Will I need hormone treatment before the implant? If yes, why? If not, why not?

Will I require external beam radiotherapy as well as brachytherapy?

How long does the procedure take? How long will I be in hospital?

How many of these procedures do you do a year?

How will I know if the implant is likely to be successful?

What are the urinary side effects? What about retention of urine?

What are your results in respect of impotence, fertility and incontinence?

Will I have much pain after the implant?

Do I have a follow-up appointment after discharge, and when will the PSA first be measured?

Ongoing how often will my PSA be checked? How will I be followed up long term?

What should the PSA be after brachytherapy? What would it mean if it doesn't reach that level? What would you do then?

What are the rectal side effects?

What if I have had previous prostate surgery, TURP or bladder neck incision?

Should the cancer return at a later date what salvage treatment options would I have?

Summary – LDR Brachytherapy

Low dose rate brachytherapy involves the ultrasound and template-guided insertion of radioactive seeds into the prostate.

Typically 60 to 120 seeds are permanently inserted in the prostate with the number inserted determined by the size of the prostate and other factors.

The seeds are inserted through the skin between the scrotum and the anus using 20 or more needles via a template. Before the procedure, the specialist will plan the positioning of the seeds in the prostate to ensure all tumours are in immediate proximity to the radioactive seeds. The procedure is generally done under general anaesthetic and requires an overnight stay in hospital.

Erectile dysfunction occurs in about 20% of cases, with these responding well to Viagra or similar medication. About 10% of patients experience short-term bowel problems such as urgency and/or diarrhoea.

Some Factors in favour of LDR Brachytherapy

It's a minimally invasive one-off procedure.

It offers lower risk of impotence and bowel problems.

Patients are usually able to return to their normal activities within a few days.

Some Factors against LDR Brachytherapy

The possibility of the seeds migrating to elsewhere in the body, e.g. the lungs; or lost during urination or intercourse.

Possibility of a need to have a urinary catheter in place for up to a few weeks after the procedure (In as many as a reported 15% of cases).

Urinary urgency and increased frequency.

Greater risk of bladder problems compared with EBRT and HDR brachytherapy.

7.6. High Dose Brachytherapy

High dose rate (HDR) brachytherapy involves the short term insertion of radioactive needles or rods into the prostate gland with a repeat treatment generally done within 12 hours. HDR brachytherapy is often referred to as temporary brachytherapy due to the radiation sources only being introduced to the prostate for short periods of time. A key attribute of HDR brachytherapy is the ability to introduce the radioactive isotope into a defined area within or immediately adjacent to the cancerous growth. This lessens the radiation damage to adjacent healthy tissue.

High-dose rate (HDR) brachytherapy is when the rate of dose delivery exceeds 12 $Gy \cdot h^{-1}$ compared to a typical LDR brachytherapy dose rate of 2 $Gy \cdot h^{-1}$. In HDR brachytherapy the radioactive needles or rods are maintained in situ in the prostate gland for a few minutes at a time. Whereas LDR seed implants are usually a monotherapy (standalone therapy), HDR brachytherapy is predominantly used in conjunction with radiotherapy, with the radiotherapy preceding or following the HDR procedure. UCLA Health in the United States has treated more than 500 patients using HDR brachytherapy as a monotherapy. Their Monotherapy HDR protocol is designed to minimize side effects by giving treatment in a series of two "implant" procedures, performed approximately one week apart. Three HDR treatments ("fractions") are given with each implant so a total of six fractions complete the course of treatment. Patients are selected for this program being deemed unsuited to their more common HDR plus EBRT procedures due to their higher Gleason score (8-10), etc. Their protocols have been replicated throughout the world.

In patients in which there is strong evidence (from biopsy results) that the cancer is fully contained within the prostate and meet low risk criteria (stage T1-T2a cancer; PSA 10 ng/ml or less and a Gleason score of 6 or less) are likely to be treated with LDR brachytherapy alone (monotherapy). Typical prescription doses for monotherapy are 145 Gray for iodine^{125} and 120-125 Gray for palladium^{103}.

I-Chow Hsu, et al.,[33] of The American Brachytherapy Society's Prostate High-Dose Rate Task Group reported in August 2008, the following inclusion criteria for patient's suited to HDR brachytherapy: Stage T1-T3b and selected stage T4; with a Gleason score of 2-10; PSA with no upper limit, but clear evidence of no metastasis beyond the prostate (TxN0M0). Exclusion criteria included severe urinary obstructive symptoms, extensive TURP defect or TURP within 6 month and/or collagen vascular disease. Patients not able to lie flat or unable to undergo anaesthesia (general, spinal, epidural, or local) were also excluded. Patients with Stage T1b-T2b and Gleason score ≤ 7 and PSA ≤ 10 ng/ml were suggested to be suited to Monotherapy (HDR alone) with prescriptive doses of 10.5 Gy for each of three exposure sessions; 8.5-9.5 Gy for each of four exposures or 6.0-7.5 Gy for 6 sessions. The Task Group recommended that those receiving HDR brachytherapy as a Boost therapy to radiation therapy (EBRT; IMRT; etc.) would receive 15 Gy for a single exposure and with 36-40 Gy of x-ray therapy (XRT); 9.5-10.5 Gy for two exposures (with 40-50 Gy XRT); 5.5-7.5 Gy for three exposures (with 40-50 Gy XRT) or 4.0-6.0 Gy for 4 HDR exposures (with 36-50 Gy XRT).

The Task Force also recommended the following post treatment follow up protocol:

Serial PSA measurements – baseline at 3-6 months and then every 3-6months and/or per institutional protocol.

Quality of life assessment - Urinary, bowel and sexual function should be prospectively assessed.

Post-Treatment biopsy - Should be reserved for protocol settings or in clinical situation where salvage local therapy is being considered.

HDR brachytherapy has a few minor advantages over LDR brachytherapy, in that no radioactive sources remain in the body after treatment. Therefore, there is no radiation risk to friends or family from being in close proximity to the patient. There is no chance of passing a seed into a partner via intercourse or of migration of radioactive seeds into other organs of the body (e.g. lungs) as can occur (very infrequently) after LDR brachytherapy. The practice of HDR brachytherapy is a multi-stage procedure. It starts with the initial planning assessment in which the characteristics of the tumour are determined. The prostate is imaged via one or more modalities such as a CT scan; MRI, ultrasound or x-ray radiography. The data produced from imaging is used to create a 3D image of the tumour and its surrounding tissue. A radiation plan is then developed to determine the position of the applicators (needles or plastic catheters that contain the isotopes) to ensure no 'cold' spots or 'hot' spots in the target area. Once additional imaging has determined the correct positioning of the applicators, further aspects of the treatment plan are concluded. The images of the patient with the applicators in situ are imported into treatment planning software. The software enables multiple 2D images of the treatment site to be translated into a 3D 'virtual patient', within which the position of the applicators can be defined. The spatial relationships between the applicators, the treatment site and the surrounding healthy tissues within this 'virtual patient' are a copy of the relationships in the actual patient. The treatment planning software allows virtual radiation sources to be placed within the virtual patient. The software displays a graphical representation of the distribution of the irradiation. This allows the brachytherapy team to adjust their irradiation plan before radiation insertion begins.

The radiation sources are inserted into the applicators by a process called 'after-loading'. Today after-loading is generally achieved via an automated system that protects the clinicians from radiation exposure. This is achieved by initially housing the radioactive sources in a shielded safe. Once the applicators are correctly positioned in the patient, they are connected to a 'HDR remote after-loader' machine (containing the radioactive sources) through a series of connecting guide tubes. The treatment plan is sent to the after-loader, which then controls the delivery of the sources along the guide tubes into the pre-specified positions within the applicator. This process is fully automated which allows staff to leave the treatment room. The sources remain in place for a pre-specified length of time (usually 2 to 5 minutes), again following the treatment plan, following which they are returned along the tubes to the after-loader.

The applicators are removed and the patient is transferred to the recovery ward. If a second session is planned, the applicators and the template through which the applicators pass, is maintained in situ for the second session which is not done under anaesthetic and is painless. Generally a second session starts about 6 hours after the first session is completed. It is necessary for the patient to lie still on their back over this period to avoid moving the applicators and template in the perineum area. It is an uncomfortable and somewhat painful wait before the second (or in some instances a third) session. A Foleys catheter (for urine drainage) remains in place until the applicators and template are removed. The computer controlled system allows the clinician/radiation oncologist to control the radiation dose in different regions of the prostate. This allows the tumour to receive a higher dose with lower dosages delivered to the urethra and the area adjacent to the rectum.

The advantages of high dose brachytherapy (without follow up radiotherapy) are:

It's a minimally invasive one-off procedure

It offers lower risk of impotence, urinary incontinence and bowel problems

Patients are usually able to return to their normal activities within a few days

The ability to modify the dose after the needles are in place is a significant advantage of HDR over LDR brachytherapy.

With a follow up boost of radiotherapy, the number of sessions is generally less than for radiotherapy alone, which sees less radiation exposure to healthy tissue. In some instances in both forms of brachytherapy, the radiation oncologist may also recommend short-term hormonal ablation therapy, which begins three months before the brachytherapy and continues for 3 - 12 months afterwards. This therapy consists of a quarterly injection of Lupron® or Zoladex®, and an anti-androgen medication like Casodex®. The hormone therapy will shrink the cancer, shrink the prostate gland, and reduce the PSA level. The likely result being there will be less cancer cells for the radiation treatment to destroy.

What Questions should I ask my Specialist about HDR Brachytherapy?

The questions are general the same as for LDR Brachytherapy, but with a few exceptions.

Could my prostate be too big to do HDR brachytherapy?

Will I need hormone treatment before the implant? If yes why? If not, why not?

Will I require external beam radiotherapy as well as brachytherapy? If so, how long after the brachytherapy should radiotherapy begin? How many treatments (or fractions as they are known) of radiotherapy are needed?

How long does the brachytherapy procedure take? How long will I be in hospital?

How many of these procedures do you do a year?

How will I know if the treatment is likely to be successful?

What are the urinary side effects? What about retention of urine?

What are your results in respect of impotence, fertility and incontinence?

Will I have much pain after the implant?

Do I have a follow-up appointment after discharge, and when will the PSA first be measured?

Ongoing how often will my PSA be checked? How will I be followed up long term?

What should the PSA level be after brachytherapy? What would it mean if it doesn't reach that level? What would you do then?

What are the rectal side effects?

What if I have had previous prostate surgery, TURP or bladder neck incision?

Should the cancer return at a later date what salvage treatment options would I have?

Summary – HDR Brachytherapy

High dose rate (HDR) brachytherapy involves the short term insertion of radioactive needles or rods into the prostate gland with a repeat treatment generally done within 12 hours.

A key attribute of HDR brachytherapy is the ability to introduce the radioactive isotope into a defined area within or immediately adjacent to the cancerous growth. This lessens the radiation damage to adjacent healthy tissue.

HDR brachytherapy is predominantly used in conjunction with radiotherapy, with the radiotherapy preceding or following the HDR procedure.

Some Factors in favour of HDR Brachytherapy

No radioactive source remains in the body after the procedure is completed.

As a monotherapy, it offers the shortest course of treatment.

As a combined therapy, a shorter course of EBRT (or similar) is required before or generally after the procedure.

Provides excellent radiation coverage of any microscopic extension of the cancer immediately beyond the prostate.

Minimizes areas of radiation overdose (hot spots) or underdose (cold spots) within the prostate.

A key advantage of combined HDR brachytherapy over a course of EBRT without HDR, is it offers superior control of the distribution of radiation within and around the prostate.

Radiation control rates are correspondingly high and complication rates low with HDR brachytherapy.

As a monotherapy, it is used as a salvage treatment after cancer recurrence.

Some Factors against HDR Brachytherapy

Between 50% and 67% of patients experience dysuria, urinary urgency and/or urinary retention. These conditions generally reduce over time sometimes needing medicinal support.

Erectile dysfunction has been reported in 16% of cases.

Urinary stress incontinence and urethral stricture has been reported in less than 5% of HDR monotherapy cases.

Unsuitable for men with a prostate volume of more than 60 ml due to the physical inability to reach all affected areas.

Chapter 8.

Hyperthermia

The ancient Greeks treated sick patients with heat. In 500BC, Parminides, a Greek physician was purported to say, *"Give me a chance to create a fever, and I will cure any disease"*. The Egyptians were said to have treated tumours with heat as early as 5000 BC. There are documented occasions where cancer patients who have been subjected to prolonged high fever due to being stricken with an infectious disease, have seen their cancer regress as a result of being exposed to higher than normal body temperatures.

Hyperthermia (also called thermotherapy) is a type of cancer treatment in which body tissue is exposed to high temperatures. Research has shown that elevated temperatures of between 39° C (102° F) and 48° C (118° F) can damage and kill cancer cells, usually with minimal injury to normal tissues. Hyperthermia treatment, when combined with other treatments such as chemotherapy or radiation, usually leads to a significant reduction in tumour size. Some hyperthermia treatments in themselves lead to good treatment outcomes. Other than for some prostate cancer treatment regimens, hyperthermia is usually non-invasive. There are two broad forms of hyperthermia treatment: whole body hyperthermia and local or regional hyperthermia. Both techniques have been practiced in a number of European clinics for more than 20 years, with patients travelling from all over the world to undergo treatment. It is used for treating several types of cancer such as prostate, breast, throat, tongue, etc.

Whole body hyperthermia (WBH)

This form of treatment sees the whole body (except for the head) being subjected to a higher than normal body temperature. It is often used in patients where metastases have taken hold with secondary cancers appearing in the lymph glands or other organs. Changes take place in body cells when they are exposed to higher-than-normal body temperatures. These higher temperatures see the "elevation" of heat shock proteins from the cancer cells, which allow the body's own immune system to better see these cancerous cells and attack them. This "elevation" of heat shock proteins, also allows lower doses of chemotherapy or radiation to kill these cancer cells.

In whole body hyperthermia, the heating is accurately controlled and is provided by either microwave or infrared energy. The patient might be treated for one to several hours at a time with two, three or four follow-up treatments being planned over a ten day or longer period. It is usual that the patient also receives an adjutant treatment such as chemotherapy during, or after the whole body hyperthermia treatment. This form of treatment usually sees temperatures limited to a maximum of 42° C (108° F). In Europe, the method of heating is almost exclusively via infrared, for a number of reasons:

Infrared units (special LED radiators deliver computer-generated water-filtered IR – A type wavelengths that penetrate the skin to deliver heat to the capillary bed) have been found to preferentially stimulate the immune system, whereas microwave units do not obtain an immune response

They do not develop hot spots or burn the patient as is possible with microwave devices.

Radiation treatment after hyperthermia also yields good outcomes, but chemotherapy appears to yield the best results. Research has shown that WBH can have a significant beneficial effect on the immune function of an organism infected with cancer. The introduction of infrared A-type generated heat, sees the tumour go into apoptosis (cell death). This is achieved by metabolic exhaustion, loss of ATP production, hypoxemia, an increase in lactic acid and the production of heat shock proteins. The surrounding healthy tissue is actually improved by WBH due to better oxidation, higher production of ATP, higher blood flow, and the increase and activation of immune cells.[1]

More generally, WBH is often used as a treatment of last resort. The German clinics offer an integrative approach to treatment and have achieved excellent results. The protocol used at the St Georg Clinic, near Munich, Germany, sees the body heated to 41.6-41.8° C (107° F)

for 90 minutes. A temporary state of hyperglycaemia, using glucose, is induced in the patient to improve tumour response. Low-dose chemotherapy and/or natural therapies such as intravenous vitamin C (25-50 grams) are administered. The resultant high acidity and hypoxia damage the blood vessels that feed the cancer cells and WBH damages the membranes, proteins and enzymes of the cancer cells, thus leaving them more vulnerable to attack by the anticancer agents that have been introduced.

WBH is still considered as an experimental treatment in many countries, including the USA. Converse to this, is the fact that the treatment is covered by health insurance policies in Germany.

Local and Regional Hyperthermia

Local or regional hyperthermia is the use of heat applied directly to an area of the body, usually the cancer tumour. This kind of hyperthermia has been used alone or in combination with such therapies as chemotherapy and radiation, to treat a wide variety of cancers including prostate cancer, with excellent results. These cancers include melanomas, oesophageal or stomach cancers, pancreatic cancers, sarcomas, bone tumours, cervical cancers, head and neck cancers, and rectal cancers. Hyperthermia causes direct cytotoxicity in the tumour, enhances its sensitivity to radiation, and improves the effectiveness of many chemotherapeutic agents in sometimes drug-resistant cells.[2]

The heat is generated by radio frequency, microwave, ultrasound, or magnetic energy. The heat is applied to the body surface, inside body cavities or into deep body tissue via the use of needles or probes. Local hyperthermia is used to treat a small body area or a small organ which contains one or more tumours, such as prostate cancer. When it is used to heat a larger part of the body, such as an entire limb or larger organs, it is referred to as regional hyperthermia.

In 2011, the US Food and Drug Administration approved the first RF device (the BSD 2000 from the BSD Medical Corporation, Salt Lake City, Utah, USA) for the treatment of cervical cancer to be followed by radiation treatment. The BSD-2000 Hyperthermia System is intended to deliver focused therapeutic heating (hyperthermia) at temperatures greater than 40° C (104° F) to cancerous tumours. It applies radiofrequency (RF) energy at the frequency range of 75 to 120 mHz. (The term RF energy is a general term that refers to frequencies of the spectrum above audio and below that of light). The BSD-2000 delivers RF energy to a patient using a power source and an array of antennae that surround the patient's body. The energy delivered by the device can be electronically focused to produce a localized EM power field. This can be adjusted to target the 3-dimensional shape, size, and location of the tumour, providing dynamic control of the heat delivered to the tumour region. This method of therapeutic heating utilizes the adjustment of frequency, phase, and amplitude from multiple power sources, along with the selection of an appropriate applicator and careful patient positioning, to optimize heating of the targeted body tissues. (In the USA, the BSD- 2000 has a Humanitarian Device Exemption (HDE) approval for use in conjunction with radiation therapy in the treatment of cervical carcinoma patients. These women would normally be treated with combined chemotherapy and radiation, but are ineligible for chemotherapy due to patient related factors). BSD previously obtained FDA approval for their microwave energy-driven (915 mHz) BSD 500 device which is now approved for stand-alone treatment, or to be used in conjunction with radiation therapy. This portable unit is used to treat solid cancers (including adenocarcinoma) in surface or sub-surface situations via superficial or interstitial (internal) applicators. It is often used with recurrent cancers and is also used in conjunction with brachytherapy procedures.

Further details on non-local hyperthermia are accessible via Appendix 3.

An Australian and similar clinics in Austria, Belgium, Canada, China, Denmark, Germany, Greece, Hungary, Israel, Italy, Jordan, Romania, Russia, South Korea, The Netherlands, Turkey and Ukraine offer cancer treatment using one of the loco-regional Oncotherm systems. These clinics have treated more than 150,000 cancer patients over the last 20 years. The first oncothermia clinic in Australia opened at the Prince of Wales Hospital in 2012.

Local hyperthermia usually targets a small area such as the tumour itself. The tumour is accessed directly via needles or probes and is referred to as interstitial hyperthermia. The low blood flow in cancerous cells, contributes to their rapid temperature increase under hyperthermia conditions, whereas the healthy cells adjacent to the tumour have normal blood flow that rapidly dissipates the heat build-up. Thus, a temperature gradient is created between the cancer cells and the normal cells. The tumour mass becomes inactive at 42° C (108° F) or higher temperatures. The temperature of the healthy cells is limited to a maximum of about 40° C (104° F), by the cooling effects of normal blood flow. They are not adversely affected by the induced heat.

The heating of the cancer cells also leads to the release of heat shock proteins (HSPs) by the cancer cells. HSPs are found in almost all living organisms, from bacteria to humans and when subjected to heat shock as they are in hyperthermia, their expression is increased (or in illustrative terms, they put up a flag which says "here I am, come and get me"). This action 'allows' the cancer cells to be identified by the body's immune system and makes them far more vulnerable to attack by one's own immune system, radiation and by low dose chemical or biological agents. Therefore, hyperthermia is usually used in conjunction with one of these main stream therapies.

Local hyperthermia kills cancer cells by:

Tissue acidosis (as cells become more acidic, they become more heat-sensitive).

Damage to poorly developed blood capillaries.

Damage to tumour cell membranes, proteins and enzymes

Cellular repair mechanism failure.

DNA and RNA synthesis changes.

Failure of antioxidant systems.

Impact on heat shock proteins (HSP), which are made more "visible" to the body's immune mechanisms.

A number of different modalities exist for localized hyperthermia. These include: thermo-radiotherapy; microwave hyperthermia; transrectal ultrasound; radiofrequency interstitial tumour ablation; transrectal hyperthermia; thermo-immunotherapy and transurethral hyperthermia (TUH). These were reviewed in a paper by Douwes and Lieberman, published in the June 2002 issue of Alternative & Complementary Therapies.[3] This latter paper focussed in the main on transurethral hyperthermia (TUH) which is a speciality of Dr Douwes's Clinic St. Georg in Germany. They have successfully treated many hundreds of early stage prostate cancer sufferers over more than 20 years. They also treat advanced prostate cancer cases using whole body hyperthermia with adjuvant chemotherapy or conformal radiation treatment.

TUH treatment introduces the RF generated heat, via a thin probe inserted into the prostate via the urethra and penis. This probe also includes a temperature sensor that is used to very precisely control the procedure. The Douwes TUH protocol sees the prostate temperature raised to 47 - 49° C (117 - 120° F) and maintained in this range for up to 60 minutes. Research has shown that the optimum "killing" temperature is at or above 43° C (109° F) and that time duration and temperature optimize hyperthermia treatment.[4,5,6] Two or three treatments over a week appear to be their norm. Generally, they also treat patients with large doses of vitamin C and other complementary anti-cancer agents during the outpatient visits to the clinic. The medical professionalism and proficiency in hyperthermia-centred cancer treatment of the three or four German clinics offering hyperthermia treatment is well-established and they treat large numbers of patients from all over the world.

One issue that might be of concern to prostate cancer sufferers is the absence of clinics outside of Germany and Austria that use TUH therapy. I asked a manufacturer of a temperature-based prostate cancer therapy as to why there we not TUH clinics everywhere. His response was that local hyperthermia had one drawback. This was that cancer cells immediately adjacent to normal blood pathways were able to dissipate the induced heat before cell apoptosis took place. A likely response from the clinics using TUH would be that the temperature elevation and its duration are sufficient to achieve cell apoptosis. It also ensures that the heat shock proteins are activated making the cancer cells susceptible to attack by the body's own immune system and the chemical and biological agents introduced during the TUH treatment.

I recently became aware of another hyperthermia type technology called **Low Dose Alternating Current (LDAC)** technology. This patented system from LaZure Scientific Inc., has just started being used in very limited human trials in Europe. LDAC operates by the introduction of 'probes' into the prostate via a system similar to that use to insert LDR brachytherapy seeds. LDAC delivers a precisely controlled electric field throughout the entire prostate that impacts all cells in the gland simultaneously. They have found that cancer cells are more susceptible to the electric field than normal cells in the same space. Their unique system provides for the most controlled delivery of electric fields and heat. Each electrode within the prostate is monitoring electrical properties and heat to ensure that at every location, the maximum possible field is being delivered at all times without causing burning within the space being treated. The evolution of LDAC will be interesting to watch as it develops over the next few years.

Summary – Hyperthermia

Hyperthermia is a type of cancer treatment in which body tissue is exposed to temperatures of between 39° C (102° F) and 48° C (118° F) for sustained periods. This practice damages and kills cancer cells, usually with minimal injury to normal tissues.

At these temperatures, heat shock proteins become more "visible" to the body's immune system and the cancer cells are more vulnerable to attack by low dose chemotherapy or other biological agents.

The Douwes local transurethral hyperthermia (TUH) protocol sees the prostate temperature raised to between 47 and 49° C (117 - 120° F) and maintained in this range for up to 60 minutes. The heating is radiofrequency induced and is precisely monitored and controlled. For TUH, the optimum "killing" temperature is considered to be at or above 43° C (109° F) with both time duration and temperature considered important.

Best results are obtained when the TUH protocol is used in conjunction with a complete androgen blockage (treatment with gonadotropin-releasing hormone).

Whole body hyperthermia is used in many countries to treat metastatic cancers.

Some Factors in favour of TUH

It is a simple, low cost procedure.

It causes direct cytotoxicity (cell death) in cancer cells and makes them additionally susceptible to chemotherapeutic and biological agents.

Some Factors against TUH

Radiofrequency local TUH is only available from clinics in Germany and Austria.

Small possibility of the survival of some cancer cells that are immediately adjacent to normal blood supply vessels. (The desired "killing" temperature is not achieved for the required duration due to the heat removal by the blood supply).The simultaneous use of biological and chemotherapeutical agents is used together with the enhanced immune system of the body, to destroy these remaining cancer cells.

The US FDA has approved microwave-induced hyperthermia only when it is used in conjunction with radiation treatment.

Chapter 9.

Cryotherapy

Cryotherapy is also known as cryosurgery or cryoablation. It is a procedure in which cancer cells are killed by freezing them by surrounding them with ice crystals. Tiny needles are inserted into the prostate under TRUS (transrectal ultrasound) guidance. Argon and helium gases are introduced sequentially via these needles into the cancerous zones of the prostate which provide a cooling and subsequent heating cycle. The urethra, which goes through the penis and through the centre of the prostate, is protected by a heated catheter to protect it against freezing and resultant damage. The American Urological Association recently issued Best Practice Guidelines for the use of cryosurgery for the treatment of prostate cancer.[1] It provides considerable information on cryosurgery and I consider it essential reading for anyone contemplating cryotherapy, either as an initial treatment or as a salvage treatment after biochemical recurrence of the disease. Refer to the Appendix 3 for their web site details.

Cryotherapy is generally used in patients with low-risk tumours. PSA levels less than 10 ng/ml, Gleason score lower than 7, and Stage T1c or T2a, and some say, even up to T3a. The risk of temporary or permanent impotence after the procedure is significant which considerably reduces the number of men undergoing cryotherapy. It is also an alternative procedure for patients who have had cancer return after radiation therapy.[2] It has a part to play in cases where the cancer has spread just beyond the prostate. Cryotherapy is unlikely to be recommended for men who have a very large prostate due to the difficulty in freezing larger areas whilst containing the freezing to tissue adjacent to the prostate.

This form of prostate treatment started in the 60's, but went into decline due to relatively poor outcomes being achieved. At that time liquid nitrogen was used as the coolant. The technique re-surfaced again in 1993, after significant improvements in the available equipment, a change to argon and helium gases and TURP guidance becoming possible. Due to the selectivity of patients suited to cryotherapy and the relatively small number of patients undergoing the technique, few long-term studies appear to have been done to prove it efficacy, etc. One study by D. Bahn, et al., published in 2002, reported on the seven year outcomes of 593 patients treated with cryoablation as the primary prostate cancer treatment. The study concluded that no serious complications were observed and that *"cryoablation was shown to equal or surpass the outcome data of external-beam radiation, 3-dimensional conformal radiation, and brachytherapy. The 7-year outcome data provide compelling validation of TCAP (the cryoablation of the prostate) as an efficacious treatment modality for locally confined and locally advanced prostatic carcinoma".* However, the study revealed almost 95% of men who were potent before the treatment, were impotent after cryoablation. The remaining 5% regained their erectile function an average of 16.4 months after treatment. For those with normal urinary control before the procedure, the incontinence rate was 84% post treatment, with an average 6.1 months post treatment recovery time.[3] Since this study was concluded, there have been considerable improvements in the thermal equipment used and the capability via advanced imaging techniques to more accurately "see" the areas to be ablated. Today, some urologists may have patient specific reasons for recommending this technique which from more recent studies undertaken, suggest it is a safe and effective treatment.

Serious risks are:

Erectile dysfunction (impotence) for > 80% of men, which is usually permanent, dependant on the extent of the ablation and the technique used.

Urinary incontinence is rare; (except in cases of cancer recovery treatment after prior radiation therapy).

Fistula (an abnormal opening) between the rectum and bladder is a rare complication with newer systems.

Generally temporary conditions are:

Bleeding or blood in the urine

Soreness or swelling in the region where the needles are placed

Swelling around the penis or scrotum

Pain and burning sensations in the bladder/intestinal region

Urge to empty the bladder and bowels more often (most men recover normal function in several weeks).

The urologist usually provides a pre-procedure information sheet that advises the patient what to do before the procedure as regards existing medication being taken, bowel emptying regime, etc.

Today, the procedure is generally done as an outpatient procedure (or 24 hour hospital stay) under regional (epidural) or general anaesthetic. A catheter is placed via the penis into the bladder and the bladder filled with a saline solution. A warm liquid will be passed through this catheter during the freezing stage of the procedure to ensure the urethra is protected from the freezing. The urologist will insert the needles (often called cryoprobes) and temperature sensors through the perineum area between the anus and the scrotum via a template insertion grid. Their positioning is usually assisted by a TURP-generated ultrasound image. Liquid argon gas is then passed into the needles which see the cancerous prostate tumour quickly frozen. The temperature probes monitor the temperature of the neurovascular bundles, the apex, the Denonvilliers' fascia area and external sphincter. The tissue being treated is held in this frozen state for a few minutes, before it is thawed by the introduction of helium through the needle probes.

On occasion, the urologist may decide to repeat this cycle. This is done more often than not when the treatment is a salvage procedure by ablating the posterior area of the prostate during the first freezing cycle followed by the anterior area during a second cycle. The needles are withdrawn, but the catheter is left in place for one to two weeks whilst the prostate gland heals and all swelling disappears. Impotence (erectile dysfunction) will occur in most men who have this treatment due to nerve damage caused by the freezing process.

The new SeedNet Gold™ cryotherapy system is the latest innovation from Galil Medical Inc. It offers urologists a comprehensive minimally invasive solution to treat prostate and renal cancers. SeedNet Gold™ has apparently gained wide acceptance by urologists due to its ease of use and controllability. Professor John Kearsley, Director of the Prostate Cancer Institute, St George Hospital, Sydney, Australia, said in 2013, *"the Prostate Cancer Institute will be the first centre in Australia to introduce regular cryotherapy treatment for prostate cancer, which makes us the only public institution in Australia capable of providing all treatment options for prostate cancer".* (Author's note: Proton Beam Therapy is not yet available in Australia).

"Today, minimally invasive treatments are in demand. When used in combination with extremely low/sub-zero temperatures and image monitoring, the cryotherapy system is a safe, effective and minimally invasive treatment for prostate cancer," he concluded.[4]

In a report where men had a half prostate ablation using cryotherapy in 55 men with at least one year follow-up, 95% had stable PSAs and 86% remained potent, despite 29 of the men being of medium or high risk of a recurrence. Seven men had to be retreated due to cancer developing in the other half of the prostate that was not subject to ablation. Of the 54 men without previous surgery or radiation treatment, all were continent. The authors of this research, G.Onik, et al, concluded that their *"preliminary results showed that a 'male lumpectomy' – in which the cancer region itself was destroyed – preserved potency in most patients and limits other complications (particularly incontinence) whilst maintaining good cancer control."*[5] You will have noticed that there is a huge variance in incontinence and impotence levels reported between the Bahn study (reported on earlier in this chapter) and the Onik study. The latter study focussed on the cryoablation of a specific tumour, with large areas of the prostate being unaffected, thus maintaining their function. The high potency rate (84%) and 100% continence level achieved, suggests there was no damage to the neurovascular bundles in most cases. Certainly the future of cryotherapy is in using the latest technology that allows only part of the prostate (tumour only) to be ablated, with a strong likelihood of potency and continence being retained. A recently improved FDA-approved urethral warming device has minimized urethral complications. However, all cryoablation patients need urethral catheterisation for 5 to 15 days or in rare cases for even longer, after undergoing cryotherapy.

Focal cryotherapy with its smaller needles and advanced temperature control will undoubtedly benefit from the non-invasive qualities of mpMRI and Colour Doppler ultrasound to confirm the size, shape, location and density of solid adenocarcinomas in the prostate.

Better spacing of the probes now contributes to the effectiveness and safety of the procedure.

Summary – Cryotherapy

Cryotherapy for prostate cancer until recent years presented patients with almost certain impotence.

Recent technological advances have allowed the technique to find more widespread use as a focussed procedure where individual tumours are ablated with minimal damage to healthy tissue of the prostate, rectum and surroundings.

It is used as a salvage technique for many radiation patients who have had a recurrence of their cancer.

Some Factors in Favour of Cryotherapy

It is suitable for patients regardless of their Gleason score.

It is a minimally invasive outpatient procedure that yields good outcomes in the hands of a surgeon well experienced in the technique.

It can provide an adequate margin around the tumour and can treat areas immediately external of the prostate.

If there is a recurrence of the cancer, the procedure can be repeated or radiation therapy, chemotherapy or a prostatectomy can be done.

It is suitable for many men who have prostate cancer that is resistant to radiation, hormone therapy or chemotherapy.

It is generally one of the lowest cost interventional treatments for prostate cancer.

Some Factors against Cryotherapy

It requires extensive experience and training by the surgeon. Make sure your surgeon has done many such procedures and that the procedure is not done as a "training" exercise.

It generally requires use of catheterisation for some days due to the swelling of the prostate.

Long term studies using the more recent equipment have not been concluded to date.

Chapter 10.
High Intensity Focussed Ultrasound

High Intensity Focussed Ultrasound is usually referred to as HIFU. This technique has been around since the late 1990's with two competing brands dominating the market: the Sonablate 500® from SonaCare Medical LLC, USA and the Ablatherm® from EDAP TMS S.A., Lyon, France. The latter is widely used in Europe and has subsidiaries in Italy, Germany, USA, Japan, Korea and Malaysia. The Sonablate 500® is used mainly in Japan, Australia and other countries. The technique involves heating the prostate via an ultrasonic probe placed in the rectum. At the point of focus, the tissue heats up to 70° to 90° C (158° to 194° F) and this results in the tissue dying of coagulation necrosis - (blood clotting and localised death of living cells). It is completed in a couple of hours and outcomes are generally excellent.

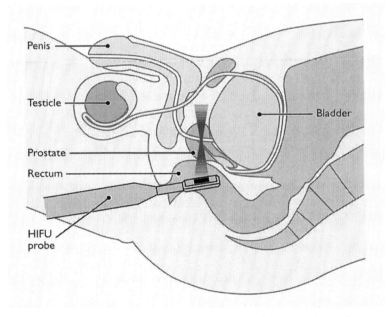

Image: Courtesy of Orchid Cancer, St Bartholomew's Hospital, London

The robotic HIFU probe is inserted into the rectum under anaesthesia. A crystal within the probe vibrates at a specific frequency when an electric current passes through it, and this produces ultrasound waves. The ultrasound waves pass through body tissue and some of the waves are reflected back to the crystal that produce an image of the prostate and its surrounding structures on a screen, which can be viewed by the urologist. By increasing the intensity of the ultrasound waves and focusing the waves on a single point (like a magnifying lens), high energy is delivered to the prostate tissue, releasing heat that causes permanent tissue ablation (cell death) of the prostate cancer. Dead tissue is passed out of the prostate with urine.

HIFU presents very manageable short term complications with possible long term complications being urethral stricture risk (9%), which may require urethral dilation or incision, stress incontinence (4%), urinary incontinence (12%), erectile dysfunction. The International Index Erectile Function (IIEF) showed overall sexual activity reduced by 20%, and specific erectile function reduced by 25% at 6-12 months after HIFU. The risks of HIFU compare favourably with Robotic/Radical Prostatectomy and are generally comparable to Brachytherapy/Radiation Therapy. Perhaps a more important measure is the recurrence rate of prostate cancer across the spectrum of available treatments. There is no standardised definition of what is a biochemical recurrence or failure that covers the various treatment types available. The Prostate Cancer Research Institute in the USA, in their PCRI Insights publication (March 2011, Vol. 14: No 1) attempt to "standardise" a definition and include a table of comparable disease free periods reported in key scientific studies covering the four common treatments: (HIFU; HDR brachytherapy + IMRT; Cryotherapy; Prostatectomy).[1,2,3]

In many instances, low or intermediate risk prostate cancer patients, have their prostate cancer confined to one lobe (or part of one lobe) of the prostate. In these instances, focal HIFU treats only the side or area of prostate proven to have cancer. This is referred to as hemi ablation or TFT (Targeted Focal Therapy). This provides the patient with less risk of erectile dysfunction, incontinence, etc., as well as good early cancer control. The Lancet, probably the most authoritative medical journal in the world, published the results of a study by Hashim U. Ahmed et al., which suggested that HIFU was equally suited to multifocal prostate cancer as it was to the generally more accepted unifocal cancer. The study is titled, *"Focal Therapy for Localised Unifocal and Multifocal Prostate Cancer: A Prospective Development Study."* Forty-one men were treated with focal HIFU. The follow-up period was 12 months for each patient. At that time, none were incontinent and eighty-nine percent had no impotence.[4] No histological evidence of cancer was identified in 30 of 39 men biopsied at 6 months and 36 or 92%, were free of clinically significant cancer. After re-treatment in four men, 95% had no evidence of disease on mpMRI at 12 months.

A prospective trial using HIFU hemi ablation at University College London has demonstrated feasibility, safety and encouraging functional outcomes (95% preservation of urinary/sexual function) and encouraging early cancer control (90% absence of any prostate cancer on protocol mandated biopsies).[5]

A number of scientific papers have been published over the past 5 years, which have reviewed the latest literature on the use of HIFU in a clinical setting. The two major reviews found that no randomised controlled studies appear to exist in the 30 plus studies considered by each review. The study by Cordeiro, et al.,[6] reported complications such as urinary retention, urinary tract infections, urinary incontinence and erectile dysfunction. Most patients in the study had localised prostate cancer (T1 or T2). The five year disease-free survival rate varied between 61.2% and 95%.

HIFU has been widely used in Europe, particularly for whole prostate ablation of the elderly, who may not have been able to cope well with EBRT or radical prostatectomy. A study by the Belgium KRE published in 2009, reported that an estimated 730 men being treated with HIFU in four Belgium hospitals between 2000 and 2008. A number of these patients had HIFU as a salvage treatment after a recurrence of the disease occurred. Again, this study reported the absence of randomised controlled studies and called for such studies before any possible endorsement of HIFU.[7]

HIFU and Multiparametric MRI

Multiparametric MRI is becoming an increasingly popular tool in the diagnosis of adenocarcinoma tumours of the prostate. New software has recently become available that 'merge or fuse' the imaging capability of MRI with ultrasound images. This allows real time visualization of tumours not usually seen by ultrasound. This capability offers the potential for tumours to be ablated by HIFU (or FLA) in real time under MRI imaging and control. This technology provides the capability to "destroy" the tumour alone whilst sparing healthy adjacent tissue.

In a recently published study titled: *"Image-Directed, Tissue-Preserving Focal Therapy of Prostate Cancer: a Feasibility Study of a Novel Deformable MR-US Registration System"* researchers from the University College London (UCL) investigated the feasibility of using a computer-assisted, deformable image registration software (also called fusion software). It enables 3-D, multi-parametric MRI-derived information on tumour location and size, to assist in both the planning and treatment phase of focal HIFU therapy using the Focus Surgery's Sonablate® 500 system.[8] The lead author of the study, Louise Dickinson of UCL said; *"Multi-parametric MRI has shown promise as an accurate method for determining the focality of tumours, and has promise as a potentially important enabler for minimally-invasive, tissue preserving, or focal, HIFU treatments. However, most ablative technologies for localized prostate cancer use an ultrasound platform to plan and deliver treatment, on which the tumour cannot be accurately localized. This often results in discrepancies between the tumour and target volumes, potentially leading to under-treatment at the margins, or treatment of larger tissue volumes to compensate for inaccuracies in targeting. We are very pleased that the results of this pilot study demonstrate that deformable image registration is feasible and safe when introduced into a HIFU ablative therapy setting and suggests potential for improving the accuracy of targeting lesions using a tissue-preserving focal therapy approach."* The research is based on breakthrough image analysis algorithms developed at the UCL Centre for Medical Image Computing and has undergone extensive clinical evaluation as part of clinical research studies led by Professor Mark Emberton, MD,

Professor of Interventional Oncology and Director of the Division of Surgery and Interventional Science at UCL. Twenty-six prostate cancer patients have been successfully treated at UCLH using the Sonablate® 500 with the aid of their "fusion" software as part of the INDEX Clinical Trial.

The team at UCL is now developing a commercial version of their prostate image registration/fusion software, called "SmartTarget". In early 2014, SonaCare Medical, who are a global leader in minimally-invasive HIFU technologies, and UCL Business Plc, announced a partnership to integrate SmartTarget image registration and fusion software into SonaCare Medical's innovative Sonablate® 500 HIFU system.

EDAP – TMS, the manufacturers of the Ablatherm® system, have introduced their newest HIFU product offering, this being the Focal One® Robot-Assisted Prostate Tumorectomy System. The Focal One was successfully used for its first prostate tumour removal in both France and Germany, in November 2013. By combining all the latest technologies in imaging and treatment, Focal One provides a state-of-the-art focal system with MR-fused imaging, a non-invasive surgical approach, precise and efficient therapeutic energy and end-of-treatment validation imaging capability.

One of the other focal therapies, Focus Laser Ablation, is considered in the next chapter. As HIFU and FLA are very similar techniques, many of the comments for FLA apply equally to HIFU. HIFU gets significant coverage in the European Urology Association's Guidelines on Prostate Cancer Updated April 2014 (See reference in next chapter). These guidelines include a section on complications suffered by HIFU patients. Note that the EUA and the AUA regard HIFU as an investigational technique with no HIFU devices approved for use by the FDA. Many American patients are having HIFU treatment in Bermuda, Nassau, or Toronto, Canada.[9] (The FDA are likely to make a decision on the possible approval of the Sonablate® 450 HIFU system for use as a salvage treatment after radiation therapy before the end of 2014).

The new imaging capabilities of mpMRI have been significantly enhanced by the use of image registration software (also called co-registration or fusion). It uses a complex set of computer algorithms to overlay and digitally marry two different imaging processes such as ultrasound and MRI for more complete visual information. This can be done in real time in the urologist's rooms whilst a patient is undergoing a TRUS procedure. Most proprietary or customised software has the capability of "elastically" adjusting the MRI image from point to point to get an exact match between the two image sources. This capability is called deformable or non-rigid registration and allows the combined images to be rotated in any plane. HIFU, when used with mpMRI, is likely to come into the main stream of prostate cancer therapy in coming years.

Summary – HIFU

High Intensity Focussed Ultrasound involves heating the prostate via an ultrasonic probe placed in the rectum. At the point of focus, the tissue heats up to 70° to 90° C (158° to 194° F) which results in tissue death.

The risks of HIFU compare favourably with Robotic/Radical Prostatectomy and are generally comparable to Brachytherapy/Radiation Therapy.

HIFU is equally successful in ablating the whole prostate (almost always in the very elderly); one lobe (half) of the prostate or a targeted tumour (or in a multi-tumour situation).

Fusion software is now in use that 'merges' a mpMRI image with the ultrasound image. This capability offers the potential for tumours to be ablated by HIFU (or FLA) in real time under MRI imaging and control. This is a 'game-changing' scenario which when combined with the newest HIFU systems from the two dominant manufacturers, is set to significantly increase the number of patients undergoing HIFU as a primary treatment. It also has a place in salvage treatment.

Some Factors in favour of HIFU

It is generally an outpatient procedure that allows the patient to go home after recovering from the up to three hour treatment and recovery from the anaesthetic.

It is repeatable and can be used as a primary or salvage treatment.

It does not preclude other treatments if HIFU fails.

The increase in imaging provided by mpMRI alone or when combined with a Doppler ultrasound image, allows precise ablation of individual tumours.

Some Factors against HIFU

It is still regarded as an 'investigational' technique in some jurisdictions. It is not yet approved for use by the FDA in the USA.

No randomised controlled studies exist as yet that report on longer term outcomes using mpMRI-guided HIFU ablation.

The procedure is costly in some jurisdictions with sometimes limited re-imbursement from health funds.

It is typically only used in cases with a Gleason score of 7 or less.

Chapter 11.

Focal Laser Ablation

Recent advances in multiparametric MRI (mpMRI) imaging have revolutionized the treatment of prostate cancer. More and more hospitals are upgrading their MRI facilities to incorporate a 3 Tesla mpMRI capability. In Sydney, Australia, at least four public and three private hospitals out of more than thirty now have this capability and more will join them over the next few years. Areas of the prostate that appear very suspicious for cancer on mpMRI, have provided extremely high correlation rates for cancer with targeted biopsies.[1] Some hospitals now rarely perform a random prostate biopsy without first obtaining an mpMRI.

A new treatment, Focal Laser Ablation (FLA), has begun to come into its own as a serious treatment for prostate cancer, due mainly to the impact of mpMRI. With precise mpMRI guidance it is possible to destroy small, early stage tumours using FLA. It should be noted that mpMRI really requires a 3 Tesla strength system, which provides the ability to detect even very small tumours. The earlier 1.5 T machines, even with an endorectal coil, are generally not powerful enough to get the job done properly.[2]

A 38 person sample study by David Yao, et al., reported a 6 fold increase in tumours detected by MRI-prompted biopsies compared to conventional non-focused biopsy methods. The anterior lobe and central zone, which are areas characteristically under sampled by conventional biopsies, contained a majority of these tumours. Of the tumours detected via MRI, 93% were clinically significant (≥Gleason 7 or >50% of cores were positive for cancer).[3]

Over the past several years, Dr. Dan Sperling, Medical Director and Chief of Interventional Uroradiology at the Sperling Prostate Cancer Centre in New York City, has pioneered a technique for transrectal focal ablation of prostate cancer under MRI guidance. His description of the procedure can be followed at https://www.youtube.com/watch?v=lX1d--Dx56A.

It broadly involves the following steps:

The prostate area is locally anaesthetized.

The prostate is scanned using MRI to identify the size and exact location of the tumour.

A biopsy of the tumour is taken to confirm the diagnosis. Placement of the needle is assisted by visibility on MRI.

A thin laser probe (1.6mm) is introduced into the tumour again under MRI guidance.

The laser ablation is commenced with the tumour heated to destruction within 3 minutes under carefully controlled conditions and MRI imaging.

The whole procedure, which is completely painless to the patient, is completed in about an hour, with the patient going home immediately after being de-briefed by the doctor. The protocol also calls for real time monitoring of the temperature of critical structures adjacent to the prostate (rectum, urinary sphincter and erectile nerves) to prevent collateral damage to the same. Numerous safeguards are built into the system to protect the patient during the ablation process. Dr Sperling has, up until early 2012, treated more than 100 patients and has reported no side effects being experienced by any treated patient.[4] Uptake of the FLA procedure in the USA medical centres has been reasonably slow. It recently became available in Sydney, Australia, via a medical practice associated with the Macquarie University Hospital.

Two well-respected clinical institutions, the National Cancer Institute (NCI), and the University of Chicago Medicine (UCM), have started clinical trials on Focal Laser Ablation (FLA). They are considered as interventional trials, meaning that a treatment is under investigation. The UCM Phase 1 trial reported in the June 2013 Radiology that *"Transperineal MR imaging-guided focal laser ablation appears to be a feasible and safe focal therapy option for clinically low-risk prostate cancer"*.[5] Other studies are underway in Australia and elsewhere.

Due to the newness of the FLA technique, medical centres are inclined to have an extensive post treatment surveillance protocol. One such protocol requires within 3 to 6 months of treatment:

A digital rectal examination (DRE)

A PSA test

A PCA3 Test (this requires the prostate to be massaged during the DRE)

An mpMRI-guided targeted biopsy (probably one or two needles only).

If no residual disease is present, these tests will be repeated one year later with the exception of a targeted biopsy of the region of interest and a 12 core random biopsy will be performed, both done under TRUS guidance. Thereafter, all of the tests with the exception of mpMRI, will be performed every six months. The mpMRI will be performed annually every two years.[6]

FLA is still considered in the USA and Europe as a treatment under investigation. An international multidisciplinary panel of 48 experts recently agreed on a standardised study design for future clinical trials for FLA. Their focal trial design standards were:

Patient inclusion: PSA <15 ng/ml, clinical stage T1c-T2a, Gleason 3+3 or 3+4, life expectancy >10 years, and any prostate volume

Post-treatment evaluation: TRUS biopsies taken between 6-12 months after treatment

Primary objective: focal ablation of clinically significant disease with negative biopsies at 12 months after treatment as the primary endpoint.

What is beyond belief is the absence of any reference to mpMRI in their design standards. This latter technique is rapidly revolutionising focal therapies for the treatment of prostate cancer. What can perhaps be deduced by this omission is the conservatism of many urologists, and the possible protection of "their patch" (biopsies to be done by urologists and not by radiologists)!

Who is a Candidate for Focal Laser Ablation of the Prostate?

Men are diagnosed with either unifocal or multifocal prostate cancer. Unifocal cancers exist in one lobe of the prostate only. These cancers are ablated which leaves the rest of that lobe (consisting of healthy tissue) and the other lobe unaffected by the treatment. It is obvious that the ideal candidate for this procedure is an individual who places a high priority on preserving sexual function. Further, he should have a single prostate region of interest (one prostate lobe only) as shown on the mpMRI that is confirmed by biopsy to be low or intermediate prostate cancer. Men with multifocal (both lobes) low risk cancer unrelated to a region of interest may also be possible candidates dependant on their data. The European Urology Association Guidelines on Prostate Cancer Update April 2014, include quite different selection criteria for focal therapies.[7] They also state: *"Focal therapy of any sort is investigational, and the follow-up and retreatment criteria are unclear."*

Editor Note: The above EUA Guidelines make no reference to FLA. They only refer to two foci treatments: HIFU and CSAP (Cryosurgery of the Prostate). They are very comprehensive and you might find it easier to ready the pocket version.[8]

FLA as a salvage or recurrent prostate cancer treatment

FLA is an excellent modality when combined with mpMRI for the detection and treatment of recurrent prostate cancer. All prostate cancer treatments (excluding active surveillance) see a percentage of patients go on to have a biochemical recurrence of their cancer. Even after a prostatectomy in which the entire prostate and seminal vesicles are removed, some cancer cells might remain that over time manifest themselves in the form of a continuous rise in PSA value.

It is difficult to detect recurrent tumours due to their generally small size and due to dramatic changes in the prostate itself after radiation or focal treatment. The benefit that FLA presents when used in conjunction with a 3T mpMRI system, is that the cancers can be identified and successfully ablated under MRI guidance. Side effects are generally less than those experienced with a salvage prostatectomy. Erectile dysfunction and urinary incontinence are rarely experienced when the procedure is undertaken by an experienced surgeon who has performed many such FLA and mpMRI salvage procedures. The salvage procedure that is generally followed is similar to that which would be undertaken during an initial diagnosis and treatment using FLA with mpMRI:

mpMRI scan identifies any areas of interest.

An MRI targeted biopsy or TRUS guided biopsy using computer co-registration is performed to confirm that the region/s of interest is/are cancerous.

A 3D Colour Doppler Ultrasound is also usually done to evaluate blood flow in the tumour area; tumour volume, size, tissue density and exact shape; location of the neurovascular bundles, etc.

The tumour/s located is/are ablated under MRI guidance. A small safety margin external of the tumour is also ablated.

Should a biopsy be done prior to the mpMRI scan, the alignment of the cancer in the biopsy cores is checked against the areas of interest identified by the mpMRI scan. A good match confirms prostate cancer at that location. FLA when used with mpMRI is likely to come into the main stream of prostate cancer therapy in coming years.

Summary – FLA

Probably the newest approved treatment for prostate cancer. FLA has begun to come into its own as a serious treatment, due mainly to the impact of mpMRI imaging. Its impact for the detection of tumours and then guidance in their destruction via FLA (or HIFU) is very significant.

FLA takes full advantage of the significantly higher detection level of tumours by MRI targeted biopsies compared with standard biopsy methods.

Individuals who places a high priority on preserving sexual function should seriously consider FLA under MRI guidance

Focal therapy of any sort is still regarded as investigational.

The technique is becoming more and more a treatment of choice demanded by patients. The urology profession are responding to this demand with more centres starting to offer this method of treatment.

Some Factors in favour of FLA

It is minimally invasive, with patients feeling no pain and go home shortly after the one hour procedure is completed.

Patients generally maintain a high degree of sexual function and incontinence is uncommon.

It can be used as a primary or salvage treatment. It does not limit re-treatment with FLA or any other treatment protocol should the cancer progress elsewhere in the prostate.

Some Factors against FLA

Whilst now extensively available in the USA, FLA of the prostate is still not FDA approved and some health funds do not fully cover the procedure.

With any new technique, it takes time for long term data to become available to conclusively prove the viability of the methodology. This, coupled with the general conservatism of the urology profession, delays the widespread uptake of techniques like FLA combined with mpMRI.

Possible inexperience of urologists in mastering the technique.

It is generally suitable for low and intermediate risk patients only.

Chapter 12.

Hormone Therapy

It has long been known that testosterone, a male hormone that is produced by the testicles, is involved in stimulating the further development of cancer cells in the prostate after the cancer has started. Before looking at the various hormone therapy options, let's look at few definitions and statements that will make the treatments outlined more understandable:

Hormones are biochemical substances that are made in glands in the body. They affect the action of cells and tissue in the human body and reach their target areas mainly via the bloodstream.

Androgens are male sex hormones and are a class of hormones that control the development and maintenance of male characteristics.

Testosterone and dihydrotestosterone (DHT) are the two most abundant androgens in men. Almost all testosterone is produced in the testicles; a small amount is produced by the adrenal glands. Prostate cancer cells also have the ability to produce testosterone.

Hormone therapy, also called androgen deprivation therapy (ADT) or androgen suppression therapy (AST) is a powerful form of anti-cancer treatment in that it inhibits the production of androgens, blocks androgen action, or both. Hormone therapy can slow prostate cancer cell growth, which is stimulated by androgens. Androgens are necessary for normal growth and function of the prostate. They are also necessary for the growth of prostate cancer cells.

Early in their development, prostate cancers need relatively high levels of androgens (mainly testosterone and DHT) to grow. Such prostate cancers are referred to as androgen dependent or androgen sensitive because treatments that decrease androgen levels or block androgen activity can inhibit their growth. Current hormone therapy treatments do one of three things:

They block the *production* of androgens throughout the body

They block *the action* of androgens in the body

They *reduce* androgen production by the testicles.

Treatments that reduce androgen production by the testicles are the most commonly used hormone therapies for prostate cancer. These include:

Orchiectomy is a surgical procedure to remove both testicles, in cases of prostate cancer. This radical treatment is called surgical castration and is permanent and irreversible. The level of testosterone in the blood usually drops to about 10% of the previous level after the surgery. It is done only occasionally today as the same outcome can be achieved biochemically.

Drugs called **luteinizing hormone-releasing hormone (LHRH) agonists**, prevent the secretion of a hormone called **luteinizing hormone**. The LHRH agonist is a drug that is usually implanted by injection under the skin. Treatment with a LHRH drug is referred to as medical castration or chemical castration. It works by lowering the androgen levels in the body to the same extent as an orchiectomy. It offers one major advantage over an orchiectomy in that its effect is reversible. Once treatment is stopped and the drug leeches out of the body, androgen production usually resumes.

What is **testosterone flare** or **tumour flare**? The LHRH drug briefly causes the pituitary gland to secrete extra luteinizing hormone, before it blocks its release. This flare in advanced prostate cancer patients can manifest itself in increased bone pain, bladder obstructions or spinal cord compression.

Names of some approved LHRH agonists are:

Goserelin - Zoladex® - (Astra-Zeneca)

Histrelin - Supprelin La®; Vantas® - (Endo Pharma.)

Leuprolide - Eligard®; Lupron® - (Sanofi-Aventis; Abbott)

Triptorelin -Trelstar® -(Actavis Pharma.)

Leuprorelin- Lupron® - (Abbott Labs, et al.)

Buserelin- SupraFact® - (Sanofi-Aventis).

LHRH and GnRH agonists are used to treat advanced prostate cancer. They are often used with other treatments, such as surgery or radiation therapy and are also used to relieve pain caused by metastatic prostate cancer.

Drugs called **LHRH antagonists**, which are another form of medical castration. LHRH antagonists (sometimes called gonadotropin-releasing hormone or GnRH antagonists) work by preventing LHRH from binding to its receptors in the pituitary gland. This action stops the secretion of luteinizing hormone, which cause the body's androgen levels to drop to orchiectomy levels. LHRH antagonists are often preferred to LHRH agonists in advanced prostate cancer patients as they do not cause a testosterone flare. One LHRH antagonist, degarelix (Brand Name Firmagon® – Ferring Pharma.), was approved in late 2008 to treat advanced prostate cancer in the United States. It is given by injection.

Estrogens are hormones that promote female sex characteristics. They are able to inhibit androgen production by the testicles, but are seldom used today for prostate cancer because of their side effects and the better efficacy of other drugs.

Treatments that block the action of androgens in the body include:

Anti-androgens are drugs that compete with androgens for binding to the androgen receptor. They reduce the ability of androgens to promote prostate cancer cell growth. As anti-androgens do not block androgen production, they are mainly used in combination with orchiectomy or an LHRH agonist. Use of an anti-androgen drug in combination with orchiectomy or an LHRH agonist is called combined androgen blockage, complete androgen blockade, or maximal androgen blockade.

Some anti-androgens that are approved in the United States to treat prostate cancer include:

Flutamide (Brand Names: Flutamin®, Eulexin®) Manufacturer: Schering-Plough

It competes with testosterone and its powerful metabolite, dihydrotestosterone (DHT) for binding to androgen receptors in the prostate gland. By doing so, it prevents them from stimulating the prostate cancer cells to grow. Apparently, it is less used now, due to its side effects.

Enzalutamide (Brand Name: Xtandi®) Manufacturers: Medivation and Astellas

This was approved as a second-line therapy for metastatic castration-resistant prostate cancer (mCRPC) treatment in August 2012. This approval needed patients to have been previously treated with docetaxel. In the clinical trial leading up to the approval of Xtandi by the FDA, 0.9% of patients taking Xtandi during the trial were reported to suffer a seizure. The withdrawal of Xtandi saw the seizures disappear. The trial reported overall median survival rate of 18.4 months on Xtandi versus 13.6 months with patients on the placebo. Clinicians are excited about the potential about this new drug class.[1] In early September 2014, the FDA approved it for use in men with metastatic CRPC who have not received chemotherapy. The approval was based on the results of the phase 3 PREVAIL trial, which ended early after outstanding results were obtained.

Bicalutamide (Brand Names: Casodex®, Cosudex®) Manufacturer: Astra-Zeneca

It was originally launched as a combination therapy for metastatic prostate cancer patients. Subsequently, it was launched as a monotherapy for earlier stage prostate cancer. Most advanced prostate cancer patients eventually become resistant to anti-androgen including bicalutamide therapy. Anti-androgens are usually taken in tablet form.

Treatments that block the production of androgens from the adrenal glands and prostate cancer cells include:

Drugs called **Androgen Synthesis Inhibitors (ASI).** They block testosterone production by inhibiting an enzyme called CYP17 (cytochrome P450 17 alpha-hydroxylase). This enzyme, which is found in all three testosterone production sources in the body (testes, adrenal glands and cancer cells), plays a key role in allowing the body to produce testosterone from cholesterol. The adrenal glands and the prostate cancer cells produce enough androgens to support ongoing cancer cell growth. The use of an ASI reduces the testosterone levels to the lowest level possible.

Approved drugs include:

Cabazitaxel (Brand Name: Jevtana®) Manufacturer: Sanofi-Aventis. It is usually prescribed together with prednisone to treat mCRPC after chemotherapy treatment withdocetaxel (Brand Names: Taxtore®, Docefrez®) Manufacturers: Sanofi-Aventis; Sun Pharma Global

Sipuleucel-T (Brand Name: Provenge®) Manufacturer: Dendreon Corporation. Sipuleucel-T was the first therapeutic cellular immunotherapy to demonstrate effectiveness in Phase 3 clinical trials by prolonging the life of patients who have advanced to the late stage of the disease with mCRPC (which is sometimes called asymptomatic, **Hormone-Refractory Prostate Cancer (HRPC)** or **Androgen Independent Prostate Cancer (AI).** It is specifically prepared using harvested dendritic cells from the patient's white blood cells, which are incubated with a two-part fusion protein. The resultant blood product is returned to the infusion centre for re-infusion into the patient. This re-infusion leads to an immune response against cancer cells carrying the PAP antigen. This very expensive treatment, outlined by Philip W. Kantoff, et al. after a Phase 3 clinical trial, was shown to prolong life with a 4.1-month improvement in median survival (25.8 months in the sipuleucel-T group verses 21.7 months in the placebo group.[2]

Abiraterone Acetate (Brand Names: Zytiga® - Janssen Biotech Inc., Abretone® – Cadilla Pharmaceuticals). It is used to prolong the life of patients with late-stage mCRPC whose prostate cancer is not responding adequately to androgen deprivation, or treatment with anti-androgens. In Phase 3 clinical trials it was found to extend patient life by 14.8 months versus 10.9 months for the placebo group.[3] It is FDA, EMA and MHRA approved. In Australia it is TGA approved and is on the Pharmaceutical Benefits Scheme when used in combination with prednisone/prednisolone. It presents a host of side effects which need careful discussion with a medical practitioner.

Other Androgen Synthesis Inhibitors

A number of other drugs are also prescribed for late stage prostate cancer treatment, such as ketoconazole and aminoglutethimide. These are sometimes referred to as second line treatments for prostate cancer as they are/were used to treat other forms of cancer.

Hormone Therapy and Side Effects

All hormone treatments for prostate cancer have side effects to a greater or lesser extent due to the reduction in male hormones in the body. These side effects are often drug specific. You should thoroughly discuss any proposed hormone therapy treatment with your medical specialist. You need to ask what side effects are likely with the treatment proposed. A different drug may present side effects that are more manageable to you whilst still providing an appropriate therapeutic performance. Side effects might include:

Erection problems (Erectile dysfunction)

Dependant on the drug used and length of time it is taken will determine, whether or not erectile dysfunction will occur, in the short term, longer term or permanently. An erection will not be possible, if you are taking luteinizing hormone (LHRH) agonists (sometimes referred to as LH blockers), such as Zoladex®, Prostap®, Lupron®, Trelstar®, etc. This is because LHRH agonists stop the production of testosterone by the testes. Once treatment ceases, erections may return over time, sometimes taking up to a year. Agonists appear to cause more erection problems than the anti-androgens such as bicalutamide and flutamide.

Hot flushes and sweating

The stopping of testosterone production by the body leads to the occurrence of bouts of hot flushes and sweating similar to that experienced by women during menopause. Should the extent and severity of these bouts become troublesome, your doctor can prescribe a drug to lessen the symptoms.

Loss of libido

Plain and simple, hormone treatment leads to a significant loss of libido (interest in sex). It cannot be fixed by a testosterone injection as the therapy is trying to starve the prostate cancer cells of access to testosterone. Taking anti-androgen drugs, like bicalutamide, make it more likely that erections and the libido are maintained.

Breast tenderness

Bicalutamide causes severe breast tenderness and some swelling when taken in high doses. Some doctors prescribe tamoxifen to reduce symptoms in severe cases. Other agonists and anti-androgens list breast soreness and swelling or growth as a potential side effect.

Testosterone flare (or tumour pain flare)

The LHRH drug briefly causes the pituitary gland to secrete extra luteinizing hormone, before it blocks its release. This flare in advanced prostate cancer patients can manifest itself in increased bone pain, bladder obstructions or spinal cord compression. Patients are often prescribed an anti-androgen when initiating a course of agonist treatment.[5]

Tiredness or weakness

There are a few things that can be done to counteract this tiredness:

Eat a healthy diet that will give you more energy

Don't push yourself too hard and reduce any exercise regimens

Get support from family and friends

Rest up when feeling tired or fatigued.

Long Term Side Effects might include:

Mood swings

It is not uncommon to start feeling depressed about your prostate cancer situation and life in general. This feeling of depression might hang around for days or be rapidly replaced by feelings of well-being. If these mood swings are severe, the matter needs to be fully discussed with your doctor.

Bone thinning

Long term suppression of testosterone often leads to a lessening in bone thickness and the possibility of an increased risk of bone fractures. This is called osteoporosis. It can be treated by your doctor who may suggest Vitamin D, calcium or a more aggressive drug treatment.

Memory changes

It is not uncommon for men to complain of a reduction in memory recall after being on hormone therapy for some months. It is also harder to concentrate and the thought process is sometimes challenged. The memory is likely to return to previous levels after the hormone therapy has stopped and the drugs having leeched out of the body. Of course, hormone replacement therapy is not an option as suppression of testosterone levels is a vital step in fighting the prostate cancer.

Increased heart attack risk

Research suggests that there is a slight increase in the risk of a heart attack in men over 65 after taking hormone suppressors for more than 6 months. For this reason, your doctor may refer you to a cardiologist before commencing a course of long term hormone treatment.

Weight gain

Some men find their weight increasing after some months on hormone therapy. The way to control this is exercise and diet. Easily written, but much harder to do in practice! Some testosterone suppressors have their own set of short and long term effects. Discuss these with your doctor.

Author's Note: The information outlined in this chapter is presented as a guide and it is no substitute for health care delivery by your medical team.

What questions should I ask my doctor about hormone therapy?

Will hormone therapy alone cure my prostate cancer?

Do I start hormone therapy straight way or could it be delayed for a while?

How long is the hormone therapy course likely to take? Is it continuous?

Are you prescribing hormone therapy as a complement to another treatment? What is this other treatment?

How might hormone therapy affect my emotions?

What about my libido?

What side effects might I expect with what you are prescribing?

Are any of the side effects likely to be permanent?

What about my ability to maintain an erection with the drug you are prescribing?

Is there treatment to restore my ability to maintain an erection during treatment or after concluding a course of hormone therapy?

How often should I have my PSA level check whilst undergoing hormone therapy?

How is the hormone therapy delivered and how often do I need to have it "topped up"?

Is it likely to affect my long term fertility?

Summary – Hormone Therapy

Hormone therapy, also called androgen deprivation therapy (ADT), is a powerful form medical castration and anti-cancer treatment in that it inhibits the production of androgens (the sex hormones), blocks androgen action, or both. Hormone therapy can slow prostate cancer cell growth, which is stimulated by androgens.

Treatments that reduce androgen production by the testicles are the most commonly used hormone therapies for prostate cancer. Drugs called luteinizing hormone-releasing hormone (LHRH) agonists, prevent the secretion of a hormone called luteinizing hormone. The most commonly used LHRH agonists are Zoladex and Lupron.

Drugs called LHRH antagonists, are another form of medical castration. LHRH antagonists (sometimes called gonadotropin-releasing hormone or GnRH antagonists) work by preventing LHRH from binding to its receptors in the pituitary gland. Firmagon® is the most common LHRH antagonist and is used in advanced cancer cases.

Anti-androgens and androgen synthesis inhibitors complete the drug arsenal to fight late stage or hormone resistant prostate cancer.

Some Factors in favour of Hormone Therapy

It can be used as a monotherapy or in combination with other treatments like radiation.

Current hormone therapy treatments block the production and the action of androgens throughout the body. They reduce androgen production by the testicles.

A host of new drugs, used individually or in combination with other drugs or treatments, are available to extend life in metastatic prostate cancer cases.

Some Factors against Hormone Therapy

Side effects from hormonal treatment include erectile dysfunction, lack of libido, breast tenderness or growth, sweating, mood swings, bone thinning, increased heart attack risk, etc.

Chapter 13.

Chemotherapy and Immunotherapy

We heard earlier that any prostate cancer diagnosed after a biopsy would either be localised (Stage T1 or T2), advanced localised (again Stage T1, but more likely to be T2) or metastatic (stage T3 or T4). Of course, the Gleason Score determined by the pathologist examining the biopsy samples, is a very important factor in evaluating the progression of the cancer. A T3 or T4 staging assessment is likely to see a Gleason Score of between 8 to 10 (however, it could be much lower), which suggests high risk cancer is present.

Author's Note: This book has been written to broadly assist fellow prostate cancer sufferers and their friends and family. It details my journey from diagnosis to a cure (or remission). It also is a compendium of notes of current and future practice in diagnosing and treating prostate cancer. It has been prepared after a very extensive search of the research literature, company product information, books on prostate cancer, anecdotal information from other prostate cancer survivors, etc. However, I am NOT a doctor or trained in medicine. <u>**THEREFORE IT IS IMPERATIVE THAT ALL WHO READ THIS BOOK, DO SO REALISING THAT ITS CONTENT IS IN NO WAY A SUBSTITUTE FOR APPROPRIATE PROFESSIONAL MEDICAL ADVICE.**</u> *The Author takes no responsibility for the accuracy or relevance of all or any specific content contained within the book whether it be stated or implied.*

If you are diagnosed with prostate cancer of any Staging or Gleason Score, it is very important for you to fully engage with your medical specialists, to finalise a treatment or active surveillance regimen, which suits your unique circumstances. It is even more important to urgently finalise a treatment regimen with your medical specialist/s if your prostate cancer is Type 3 or T4. (Active surveillance is unlikely to be an option). Your urologist is likely to refer you for a bone scan, PET/CT scan and/or a MRI scan. Dependant on the results obtained, the urologist is likely to refer you to an oncologist, a doctor who specialises in treating cancer patients. The treatment that the oncologist might prescribe would be dependent on how far the prostate cancer may have spread. Has it reached the lymph glands and/or the seminal vesicles adjacent to the prostate or has it migrated to the pelvic bones or to other organs in the body, where secondary cancers might have formed? Note that prostate cancer cells that escape from the "box", migrate in three ways: to surrounding tissue; into the lymph glands/nodes or vessels to other parts of the body (the human lymph system is another "highway" like the blood system) or via the blood stream. Any secondary cancers that form elsewhere in the body after migration from the prostate have the same characteristics of prostate cancer.[1]

A Type 4 level cancer could have spread to the bladder, rectum, vesicles, lymph nodes or pelvic bone, all of which are adjacent to the prostate. It could also have migrated to other organs of the body. Fortunately, there is a wide array of "tools" available to your medical team to treat T3 or T4 cancer. These include hormone therapy, EBRT with or without hormone therapy, chemotherapy with hormone therapy. If the cancer is found in the bone, it is possible that **bisphosphonate treatment** might be recommended. Bisphosphonates inhibit a type of bone cell that breaks down bone and reduce the pain of bone cancer. It is sometimes called diphosphonate. Commonly used bisphosphonates [2] are:

Zoledronic acid (Zometa®) - taken as an intravenous drip

Disodium pamidronate (Aredia®) - taken as an intravenous drip

Ibandronic acid or ibandronate (Bondronat®) – taken as a capsule or an intravenous drip

Sodium clodronate (Bonefos®, Clasteon®, Loron®) - taken as a tablet or capsule

The list is completed by Denosumab (Xgeva®, Prolia®).

Chemotherapy is often prescribed if hormone therapy becomes ineffective. This situation generally occurs when the cancer cells no longer need testosterone to grow. They are said to have reached a hormone resistant or hormone refractory state. Chemo, as it is referred to in short, is usually a cycle of drugs that are administered by intravenous drip as a hospital outpatient. These cycles vary, but usually extend for two or three weeks, after which the chemo is stopped for a similar length of time, to allow the normal body cells to recover from the often harsh action of the chemotherapy.

Today, there is a whole host of chemo drugs that are used to fight prostate cancer. The more modern drugs are more likely to have less unpleasant side effects and better efficacy than older drugs – they are inclined to extend life and improve lifestyle. A frequent initial chemo drug of choice is docetaxel (Taxotere® or Docecad®), usually given with the steroid drug prednisone. If this drug does not work (or becomes ineffective), a newer drug called cabazitaxel (Jevtana®) often heads the list of the next chemo drug to be tried.

Most of these drugs work by identifying fast dividing cells and attacking them. Unfortunately, the normal cells of hair follicles, the lining of the mouth and intestines and the bone marrow are also fast dividers and impacted by the drug. Side effects such as loss of hair, mouth ulceration, diarrhoea, nausea and fatigue ensue. An allergic reaction sometimes occurs in patients receiving either of these two chemo drugs. Doctors usually prescribe other medication to lessen the impact of these possible allergies or side effects.

Another drug that is relatively new to the market is radium[223] (Xofigo®) which is mainly used in bone metastatic castration-resistant prostate cancer (CRPC). During the clinical trials it was called Alpharadin, but Bayer, its manufacturer, changed its name to Xofigo after its FDA approval in May 2013. As Bayer explains, *"Xofigo is the first and only alpha particle-emitting radioactive therapeutic agent approved by the FDA that has demonstrated improvement in overall survival."* Xofigo had also shown a delay in metastasis in the recently completed successful Phase 3 trials. Therefore, this drug can specifically help patients that have CRPC and develop bone metastases (around 90% of patients show some evidence of bone metastases). *"Bone metastases can lead to an increase in frequency of skeletal events and are shown to be the main cause of morbidity and death in patients with CRPC,"* Bayer added.

The treatment of patients with metastatic cancer is a complex business. The pros and cons are best left to an oncologist to explain as each patient will display unique characteristics that need to be considered when structuring a treatment regimen.

The recent changes in therapeutic treatments for patients with metastatic castration-resistant prostate cancer (mCRPC) have questioned the detection methods being used for metastatic cancer. Oliver Sartor, et al., in their paper *"Unmet Needs in the Prediction and Detection of Metastates in Prostate Cancer"* raised some interesting questions about the drugs used for the treatment and the improved detection of metastatic prostate cancer.[3] An important study was reported on at the 2014 ASCO meeting in Chicago. The study compared androgen deprivation therapy (ADT) alone vs ADT plus docetaxel chemotherapy in men with newly diagnosed metastatic prostate cancer. The study found that overall survival was improved by about 14 months, in the combination-therapy group. With regard to the high-risk patients (those who had either four bone lesions or visceral metastases), the overall improvement in survival was 17 months. There was also a delay in time to castrate-resistant disease.[4]

Immunotherapy

Immunotherapy is a new class of cancer-fighting tools that rely on stimulation of the immune system of the body to enable them to destroy cancer cells. An excellent pictorial illustration of the path to successful immunotherapy discovery and treatment is accessible via Appendix 3. When prostate cancer continues to grow, despite the lowering of testosterone levels by hormone therapy, treatment options become more limited. Sipuleucel -T or secondary hormone therapies such as abiraterone or enzalutamide may be added to the therapy regime, and are followed by chemotherapy agents, docetaxel or cabazitaxel. Access more information via Appendix 3.

Another promising immunotherapeutical agent is PROSTVAC®, which is a therapeutic vaccine being developed by BN ImmunoTherapeutics (a subsidiary of Bavarian Nordic A/S). It has moved to a large phase III clinical trial after a randomized phase II trial involving 122 patients with metastatic CRPC showed an 8.5 month improvement in median overall survival.[5]

Numerous institutions and biotechnology companies world-wide are spending vast amounts of money to develop immuno-therapeutical treatments that promise to radically change the prostate cancer treatment landscape in coming years.

David D. Halbert, Chairman and CEO, Caris Life Sciences in a 2014 open letter to the Boston Business Journal said:

"Molecular profiling of cancer is changing the way oncologists treat patients and is ushering in a new era of personalized medicine. By identifying the key biomarkers that show an association with drug therapies, molecular profiling can assist oncologists in determining which drug(s) would most likely work for that specific cancer patient's tumour. Equally important, profiling can also help identify drugs that are unlikely to have a clinical benefit for that patient. Biomarkers are found in a cell's DNA, RNA and protein.

Caris Life Sciences is the only profiling service offering a comprehensive analysis of all relevant drug associations currently supported by strong medical evidence. Since 2006, our Caris Molecular Intelligence molecular profiling service has been the industry's leading tumour profiling service, profiling the tumours of more than 60,000 cancer patients from 59 countries, having been ordered by 6,000 oncologists from (59 Countries) around the world. The Caris' approach to profiling, which includes multiple types of tumour analysis, including DNA, offers significantly more clinical information to an oncologist looking for new options for their patient than a DNA platform alone. Our approach can analyse all of the 236 cancer genes included in the FMI report and many more. As a result, CMI can provide up to 51 potentially relevant FDA-approved drug associations. .... (irrelevant sentence omitted)............... We are proud to offer the most clinically useful cancer- profiling service currently available to help oncologists and their patients find FDA-approved drugs that may benefit them.

Cancer patients who have exhausted standard of care, or who are battling particularly rare or aggressive cancers where no standard of care exists, deserve to know they have clinically useful options available to them." Go to Appendix 3 to access more details of their profiling service. (FMI refers to a company active in the functional and molecular imaging biomarkers space called Foundation Medicine Inc. A lot more will be heard about functional and molecular imaging biomarkers over the next few years.

Caris Life Sciences® have another interesting technology called Carisome® Microvesicle Technology. This blood-based highly-reproducible technology platform has the ability to identify and characterize circulating microvesicles (cMV's) released in the blood that serve as a signalling device for various types of cancer. cMV's are sub-cellular membrane-bound vesicles, ranging from 30 to 1500 nm in size, that can be found circulating in the blood and other body fluids. They are released from various cell types, under both normal and pathological conditions, which include cancer.[6] The key attribute of the cMV's is that each population of cMV's expresses an array of proteins that reflects its cell-of-origin. The cMV's contain a "cargo" of their cell of origin, proteins and RNA, which should provide information similar to that which would be obtained from a direct tissue biopsy. Hopefully, when this research is successfully concluded after clinical trials in the future, it is likely that a "liquid biopsy" will be possible, meaning patients may be able to avoid needle biopsies.

This technology is not specifically focussed on prostate cancer, but on cancer generally. It is included to illustrate the very rapid progress that is being made in proteomics (the science of proteins) and other biomarkers.

A recent research paper by I. Giusti, et al., highlights the potential use of vesicles as prostate cancer biomarkers.[7]

Summary – Chemotherapy and Immunotherapy

Patients diagnosed with Type 3 or Type 4 prostate cancer (after a positive biopsy and positive bone scan, PET/CT scan and/or MRI scan) are likely to be referred to an oncologist with chemotherapy to be part of the treatment regime.

If the cancer is found in the bone, bisphosphonate treatment might be recommended. Bisphosphonates inhibit a type of bone cell that breaks down bone and reduce the pain of bone cancer.

Chemotherapy is often prescribed if hormone therapy becomes ineffective. This situation generally occurs when the cancer cells no longer need testosterone to grow.

A frequent initial chemo drug of choice is docetaxel usually given with the steroid drug prednisone. If this drug does not work (or becomes ineffective), a newer drug called cabazitaxel often heads the list of the next chemo drug to be tried. Newer drugs with fewer side effects continue to become available. One is radium 223 (Xofigo®) which is mainly used in bone metastatic castration-resistant prostate cancer (CRPC).

Immunotherapy is providing a new class of cancer-fighting tools that rely on stimulation of the immune system of the body to enable them to destroy cancer cells. One such agent is PROSTVAC®, which is a vaccine that has moved to a Phase 3 clinical trial after the Phase 2 trial showed 8.5 month improvement in median overall survival in metastatic CRPC patients.

Some Factors in favour of Chemotherapy and/or Immunotherapy

Chemotherapy is an essential component in the treatment of patients with metastatic cancer.

Newer drugs are extending overall survival periods in metastatic CRPC patients with fewer serious side effects being experienced.

Immunotherapy will become a very important tool in fighting metastatic cancer in future years.

Some factors against Chemotherapy and/or Immunotherapy

Even the newer drugs have lesser but sometimes still unpleasant side effects.

Chapter 14.
Complementary and Alternative Therapies

The terms "Complementary Therapies" and "Alternative Therapies" are often incorrectly used interchangeably. "Complementary Therapies" refers to those treatments that are used together with mainstream medical practice. "Alternative Therapies" refer to treatments that are outside the mainstream of conventional medical practice. Use of natural products, mainly in the form of dietary supplements including herbs or botanicals, minerals, vitamins and probiotics, maybe used as Complementary or Alternative therapies. Mind and body practices, such as meditation, etc. also have a part to play in fighting prostate cancer.

After you have been diagnosed with prostate cancer, it is amazing how you become aware of many friends, acquaintances, work colleagues and others that have, or have had, prostate cancer. There are about 600 playing members of my golf club, and as a long term member who plays twice a week, I know perhaps half of these. The majority are in the 55 plus age group. i.e. in the zone for prostate cancer. Many keep their prostate cancer circumstances to themselves, but a few were of help to me, after my prostate cancer "plight" became known to them (I didn't go out of my way to "publicise" my affliction or seek pity). Three or four underwent radical prostatectomies, one had seed brachytherapy and two more had x-ray radiation. One of the RALP patients was a surgeon. I was a little surprised that he seemed unaware of the specifics of the various radiation treatments available to him or to have considered them in any way. Perhaps it was the 'cancer anxiety factor' at play again: get rid of the danger posed by removing it immediately!

In 2012, at about the time I was diagnosed with prostate cancer, I met Peter at a social function near where I live. Peter, a US resident, who was visiting relatives in Australia at the time, had an interesting story to relate. He had previously been diagnosed with incurable prostate cancer with metastases having set in. Five years ago, the medical profession had told him that he had better get his affairs in order as he would be dead in 12 to 18 months. At about 60 years of age, Peter was not of the mindset to accept this and committed himself to finding a way to rid himself of the cancer. His online research turned up a host of sites that provided "non-mainstream" treatments for his cancer. Some of these involved complementary and alternative therapies. One of his challenges was to sort the wheat from the chaff or scientific fact from fiction. His search led him to the Prostate Forum web site of Dr Charles "Snuffy" Myers in the USA. Access it via Appendix 3.

The Forum's content is prepared by pioneering prostate cancer oncologist and prostate cancer survivor, Dr Myers. As a leading prostate cancer specialist, Snuffy Myers offers a non-biased look at all the available treatments. He makes his analyses based on the available science—period. Peter made contact with Dr Myers and visited him in Charlottesville, Virginia in, I think, 2006. Peter was provided with a host of preparations that were to be taken daily. Each year Peter made an annual visit to see Dr Myers and return with adjustments to his treatment regime. As I understand it, some part of the treatment involved taking homeopathic substances. Each year, his PSA levels dropped or held previous levels with the metastatic progression of the prostate cancer regressing. The cost of the "pills" was in excess of $25,000 a year. Rob, a golfing friend, also visited Snuffy Myers some eight or nine years ago. More on Rob in the last chapter of the book.

My brother had been diagnosed with prostate cancer some 13 years ago. He had had exposure to Chinese medicine prior to his cancer diagnosis, and decided to undertake an ongoing course of herbal treatment prescribed by his specialist (who offered conventional treatment as well as Chinese herbal solutions). After 18 months of herbal treatment, his PSA was still elevated, but was not increasing. The 55 pills he took three times a day provided by his specialist were costing $10,000 per annum. At that time he decided to take a more proactive approach to his prostate cancer treatment and moved to another urologist. In 2000, my brother came across a book titled ***"How to Fight Prostate Cancer and Win"*** by **Ron Gellatley**. This book was first published in 1998 by Cargel Press International and has since been reprinted a number of times. At the time the book was published, Ron was an accredited Naturopath, Clinical Nutritionist, Homeopath and Medical Herbalist who had been in practice for over 15 years. His PSA was 126 and sixty percent of his prostate was cancerous. The very well written book describes in great detail his plan to rid himself of prostate cancer over a six months period. His plan culminated in his PSA reducing to 0.07 at the time of his book going to press.

The starting point of Ron's determination to rid himself of the threat to his life that was presented by his prostate cancer was his unshakable belief that he would succeed in his task based on the combination of a strong positive belief and the use of appropriate nutrients. His nutrient intake included **Bovine Cartilage** and **Lactoferrin**, which he suggests are amongst the most powerful anti-cancer nutrients available. He co-operated with Ross Gardiner, who runs a natural medicines company in Australia, to see the latter come up with a new product called **"Promaxin for Men"**. In the interim, this product has been updated to **"Promaxin Ultimate"**. Promaxin Ultimate is a high-strength herbal and nutritional male support formula scientifically proven for the symptomatic relief of the symptoms associated with medically diagnosed benign prostatic hypertrophy. One of its components is **Saw Palmetto** which assists in inhibiting the conversion of testosterone to dihydrotestosterone (DHT) in the prostate. It also blocks the attachment of dihydrotestosterone to cellular binding sites, and subsequently increases the breakdown and excretion of dihydrotestosterone from the body. (Medical research suggests that DHT is involved in the progress of healthy cells to cancer cells). Further details on "Promaxin Ultimate" are available from Medicines from Nature or from their web site accessible via Appendix 3.

There are five general categories of complementary therapies. These and their sub-groupings are:

Mind, Body and Spirit

Meditation

Tai Chi

Aromatherapy

Manual and Physical Healing

Acupuncture

Massage

Exercise

Herbal Remedies

Saw Palmetto

Green Tea

Ginseng

Diet and Nutrition

Supplements

Vitamins

Minerals

Special Diets

Pharmacological and Biological agents

Homeopathy

Shark Cartilage, Bovine Cartilage

Lactoferrin, etc.

It is arguable that some of the above therapies perhaps fit better in the "Alternative Therapy" stream rather than the "Complementary Therapy" category. Let's not get too hung up on semantics and consider them as one. There are dozens and dozens of books, some of which are excellent, that give in depth discussion on the use of the above agents or treatments. This book gives a broad overview of their use rather than a detailed investigation of their therapeutic value.

The term "holistic medicine" is often referred to when considering a number of the broad grouping listed earlier. It's all a question of what is meant by the term holistic. Some people might define it strictly as complementary and alternative medicine. Others might consider it a term that refers to treating the "whole person" rather than treating a specific ailment or disease. There is not a doctor anywhere, who wouldn't promote a healthy lifestyle which might include regular exercise, good eating habits, not smoking and the management of stress. Of course, claims made by some holistic health practitioners are exaggerated and/or are not supported by the current scientific literature. It sometimes doesn't mean the claims are necessary wrong, but that science has not yet caught up with holistic medicine. The origins of some holistic therapies, goes back thousands of years. One thing that is practically certain is the fact that an increasing number of holistic treatments are becoming more common in mainstream healthcare, where they are used as an adjunct to standard medical treatment. Perhaps the correct term for joint holistic and conventional treatment is **integrative care**.

Why do some cancer sufferers turn to holistic, complementary and/or alternative treatments?

The need to do something positive themselves to improve their situation

To alleviate or reduce the pain or side effects of conventional treatment

A need to take an active role in improving their own health and wellness which might contribute to a cure alone or by using conventional medical treatment

Mainstream treatment hasn't worked or is thought by the patient, unlikely to work.

Cancer patients who choose alternative medicine instead of mainstream cancer treatments may be putting themselves at serious risk. They are ignoring or giving up the only proven methods of treating their disease. It is essential before embarking on a

complementary or alternative therapy, to thoroughly discuss these intentions with your medical team.

Many, or even most, cancer sufferers take complementary remedies with or without their doctor's knowledge or approval. Some of these can be safely used along with standard treatment to help relieve symptoms or side effects, to ease pain, and to improve quality of live. You should discuss their use with your doctors.

Mind, Body and Spirit

Meditation

The word meditation means different things to different people. However, most consider it as a mind-body process that uses concentration or reflection to relax the body and calm the mind. There are numerous forms of meditation, each offering different outcomes to the practitioner. It can be self-directed or under the control of doctors, psychiatrists, mental health workers or yoga-masters. An independent panel convened by the US National Institutes of Health found that it might be a useful complementary therapy for treating chronic pain and sleeping problems such as insomnia. Some cancer treatment centres offer meditation or relaxation therapy with conventional medical care. However, available scientific evidence does not suggest that meditation is effective in treating cancer or any other disease, but rather, it may help to improve the quality of life for people with cancer.

Tai Chi

T'ai chi, taiji or tai chi as it is referred to in English, is an internal Chinese martial art form practiced for both its defence training and its health benefits. It is also claimed to increase longevity in older people who regularly practice the art. Medical research has found evidence that t'ai chi is helpful for improving balance and for general psychological health, and that it is associated with general health benefits in older people. A comprehensive overview of the scientific literature concluded that up to 2011, t'ai chi offered no conclusive evidence of benefit for any of the other conditions researched which included cancer.[1] T'ai chi health training concentrates on relieving the physical effects of stress on the body and mind. The focus and calmness cultivated by the meditative aspect of t'ai chi is seen as necessary in maintaining optimum health (in the sense of relieving stress and maintaining homeostasis).

Aromotherapy

Aromotherapy is the use of fragrant substances, such as essential oils, that are inhaled or applied to the skin to create a feeling of well-being and good health Aromatherapy is seen by devotees as a natural way to help patients cope with stress, chronic pain, nausea, and depression and to produce a feeling of well-being. The essential oils usually used in aromatherapy might include the following oils that are produced from plants: lavender, rosemary, eucalyptus, chamomile, jasmine, peppermint, lemon and geranium. Scientific studies suggest that no conclusive evidence of benefit was apparent in preventing or treating cancer. On the other hand, proponents of aromatherapy suggest that it of use in fighting bacterial infections; in strengthening the immune system and curing a host of maladies including cancer.

Manual and Physical Healing

Acupunture

Acupuncture has been a key component of traditional Chinese medicine (TCM) for thousands of years. Today TCM is regarded as largely pseudoscience, with no valid mechanism of action for the majority of its treatments. However, there are a large number of devotees to the practice, including Western-trained doctors. The apparent effectiveness of acupuncture relies on stimulating specific acupuncture points which corrects imbalances in the flow of qi or Ch'i as it is also known (life energy or energy flow) through channels known as meridians. Singh & Ernst in their book titled ***"Trick or Treatment: Alternative Medicine on Trial"*** London: Bantam published in 2008 stated:

"Scientists are still unable to find a shred of evidence to support the existence of meridians or Ch'i". They continued: *"The traditional principles of acupuncture are deeply flawed, as there is no evidence at all to demonstrate the existence of Ch'i or meridians"* and

"Acupuncture points and meridians are not a reality, but merely the product of an ancient Chinese philosophy".

A number of systematic reviews of randomised clinical trials (RCT's) using acupuncture for cancer pain, found that the number and quality of the RCT's were too low to draw definitive conclusions or provided insufficient evidence to determine acupuncture's effectiveness in cancer pain management.[2] The literature suggests that acupuncture has its place in management of the symptoms flowing from advanced cancer and/or its treatment rather than the cancer itself.

Massage Therapy

Massage therapy includes many different techniques in which practitioners manually manipulate the soft tissues of the body. These practices are designed to relax and de-stress the recipient.

Exercise

Physical activity is important to your overall health and quality of life. Today, many medical specialists encourage their patients to be as physically active as possible during their cancer treatment. Regular exercise is likely to provide a host of benefits that might include:

Keep or improve your physical capabilities

Improve your confidence, self-esteem and emotional state

Keep muscles from wasting due to inactivity

Lower the risk of heart disease or osteoporosis

Lessen symptoms of tiredness (fatigue)

Keep your weight in check

Improve your quality of life.

Of course, some treatments, such as a radical prostatectomy, limit the patient's capability to exercise for a while. It is important to follow the medical team's directions as regards post treatment exercise.

Herbal Remedies

Saw Palmetto

Saw palmetto extract is obtained from the fruits of the saw palmetto plant (Serenoa Repens). It is said to be used by more than two million men in the USA, as a treatment to reduce the symptoms and effects of benign prostatic hyperplasia (BPH).

The berries of the saw palmetto contain chemicals, called sterols, which are thought to interfere with the ability of testosterone to cause prostate cell growth. Early studies on saw palmetto concluded that the plant extract could ease the symptoms of benign prostatic hyperplasia (BPH), or enlarged prostate, which include difficulty urinating, urine leakage and sleep deprivation due to the need to go to the bathroom several times each night. Few of these studies included a placebo control group. A number of recent clinical trials have examined the efficacy of saw palmetto versus a placebo and/or one of the two most popular drugs (finasteride - Proscar®), and (tamsulosin - Flomax®) which are prescribed for diminished urinary flow due to the narrowing of the bladder neck caused by BPH. These recent trials/studies have used more reliable methodologies, which have found that the plant extract was no better at alleviating symptoms than taking a placebo pill.[3]

The American Cancer Society is quite unequivocal about saw palmetto: *"Available scientific studies do not support claims that saw palmetto can prevent or treat prostate cancer in humans"*. Some doctors ask men having their first PSA test to go off saw palmetto prior to having the PSA test so as to establish a true baseline result. This recommendation is made as saw palmetto affects testosterone metabolism, as does finasteride. This drug does affect PSA results, but saw palmetto does not appear to do so.

Green Tea

The Chinese have been drinking green tea for 3000 years and it also has been used in a number of other Asian countries for nearly a 1000 years. In recent years, there have been a number of significant studies into green tea and its therapeutic values. Some of these studies have shown the polyphenols in green tea to act against cancer cells in cell cultures.[4] It has been postulated that epigallocatechin (EGEC) compounds in the tea may inhibit new blood vessels from forming, thus restricting cancer cell growth. The initial studies have yielded mixed results. This has prompted the FDA to review all published studies. For a number of years the FDA has been involved in a dispute with a green tea supplier. In 2011 it announced its conclusion in this matter which stated: *"Green tea may reduce the risk of breast and prostate cancer. (The) FDA does not agree that green tea may reduce the risk because there is very little scientific evidence for the claim"*.

Ginseng

There are two types of Ginseng: The Panax Ginseng and the Siberian Ginseng. Of interest to us is only the Panax Ginseng. It comes in various qualities, so only the very best grade should be considered for use. Much of this high grade Panax Ginseng is grown, under governmental control in South Korea. The various grades are usually noted on the packaging. The US Cancer Society again considered Panax Ginseng as not offering benefit in preventing or treating prostate cancer due to lack of scientific evidence. It also warns that it can be considered dangerous in high doses and may react negatively with certain medicines as well as during surgery.

Panax Ginseng was found to include two compounds that may help protect prostate health. A 2010 study found that ginsenoside Rh2 protects against the spread of prostate cancer cells in the lab. It led to cancer cell apoptosis, or the death of prostate cancer cells.[5] The second compound was 25-OCH3-PPD. It was found to prevent prostate tumours of both androgen-dependent and androgen-independent prostate cancer in a study published in 2008. Animal testing of ginseng appears to suggest it is safe as no toxicity was found.[6] Interestingly, Panax Ginseng has shown potential as a natural treatment that can be used alongside conventional prostate cancer therapies. In a June 2008 study, ginseng was found to boost the tumour-fighting effects of docetaxel and gemcitabine (Gemzar®), which are two chemotherapy drugs.[7] It is further claimed that Panax Ginseng adds to the effectiveness of radiation treatment.

Diet and Nutrition

Supplements

Beta-sitosterol

Beta-sitosterol is a chemical compound found in plants such as P. africanum, saw palmetto, and some legumes. It is plant sterol and has a similar structure to cholesterol. Sitosterols are white, waxy powders with a characteristic odour. Plant sterols including beta-sitosterol, reduce absorption of dietary cholesterol and may provide anti-tumour effects by acting on the immune and hormonal systems of the body or by directly inducing apoptosis (cell death) in tumour cells.[8] Beta-sitosterol, at appropriate concentrations (16mM), has been shown to significantly inhibit the growth of PC-3 prostate cancer cells and to induce apoptosis.[9] Beta-sitosterol ingestion decreases the levels of cell cycle regulator proteins p21 and p27 in the cancer cells and an increased production of reactive oxygen species which also assists apoptosis.

Any potential user of beta-sitosterol should discuss its use with their doctor as it can lead to:

Increased risk of the severity of coronary artery disease in men with a history of heart attack

It is not recommended for individuals with sitosterolemia, a rare inherited fat storage disease. (Also, It should not be taken by women whilst pregnant or breast feeding).

This compound is listed only to show that there are pluses and minuses for many supplements. There is often considerable marketing hype behind many such materials. Many supplements claim to assist in the fight against cancer, but few actually help in fighting prostate cancer. The American Cancer Society makes the following generic comment for many of these compounds:

"Available scientific evidence also does not support (name of compound) *effectiveness in preventing or treating cancer or any other disease"*.

It lists a host of Herbs, Vitamins and Minerals under the Complementary and Alternative Medicine section of its web site accessible via Appendix 3. Remember that supplements are supplements and they are no substitute for having a healthy and nutritious diet.

Lycopene

Lycopene is found in tomatoes and in lesser concentrations in other fruits like pink grapefruit, guavas, papaya and apricots. Tomatoes should be cooked to see the lycopene converted to its most beneficial form as a carotenoid. It is a strong antioxidant and several scientific studies have shown a lower risk of cancer amongst high consumers of lycopene.[10]

Glutamine

Many people suffering from cancer have been found to have low glutamine levels. Glutamine is often given to malnourished patients undergoing conventional cancer treatment such as radiation or chemotherapy.[11] Glutamine is present in both vegetable and animal sources such as beef, pork, poultry, cabbage, ricotta cheeses, etc. It is usual taken as a supplement in powder, tablet or capsule form. It should not be taken with hot beverages as the heat destroys glutamine. Much more research is needed to determine the efficacy of glutamine in cancer patients. It is also important that all cancer patients undergoing chemotherapy discuss their possible interest in taking glutamine with their medical practitioner before starting to take glutamine.

Vitamins

Vitamin A is a very important nutrient that assists in general cell growth and bone development in the body. It is obtained from either animal sources such as egg yolk, dairy products or fish or from compounds like beta-carotene or alpha carotene which are found in colourful vegetables and fruit including broccoli, carrots, squash, apricots and leafy greens. The carotenes, from this source, are collectively referred to as pro-vitamin A carotenoids and are converted in the body to retinol, which is a form of Vitamin A. The Vitamin A is stored in the liver for subsequent use.

The published literature suggested that vitamin A (and other retinoids) may enhance the immune system, slow tumour growth, shrink tumours, and make some cancer treatments work better.[12]

A well-balanced diet with plenty of vegetables and fresh fruits provides people with the majority of their vitamin needs.

The results of a USA randomized controlled trial published in 2012 of male physicians taking a daily 30 nutrient multivitamin, showed a small, but statistically significant, lower risk of all cancers combined followed over a 11 year period.[13]

Minerals

Selenium

Selenium is an essential trace mineral that is found in most soils around the world. It is absorbed by plants and converted to mainly selenomethione or chelated selenium. It is used by cells in the body to defend against oxidative damage; to help maintain other antioxidants in the body (such as vitamin C and glutathione); to regulate thyroid hormone function and to stimulate the immune system.

Proponents of selenium suggest that these effects may explain its anticancer activity. The recommended dietary allowance (RDA) for selenium for both men and women is 55 micrograms (mcg) per day, but higher amounts are sometimes taken to lower the risk of cancer. The FDA warns that the daily intake of selenium should not exceed 400 mcg (1000 mcg = 1 milligram) unless supervised by a doctor. A typical Western diet might contain between 50 to 150 mcg per day. Adverse effects (including brittle hair and nails, skin rash, and neurological damage) have been observed in people taking more than 900 mcg per day. Foods rich in selenium include meats (liver and kidneys), fish, cereals and whole grains, poultry and Brazil nuts. Selenium may be found in supplemental form as sodium selenite or L-selenomethionine.

Zinc

Zinc is an essential trace mineral in human nutrition and is the most abundant trace element in cells. It plays a key role in body processes such as building DNA and RNA, producing energy, regulating the immune system, and cell metabolism. It is an important antioxidant and a component of many DNA repair proteins and is considered to be especially important in the prostate, maybe protecting it from early damage that could lead to cancer. However, recent studies with prostate cancer cells in culture indicate that zinc supplementation may be less useful in treating prostate cancer than previously thought. Converse to this, Dr Emily Ho at the Linus Pauling Research Institute, Oregon State University, reports that low zinc intake may increase the risk of prostate cancer.[14]

Zinc is found in seafood, meats, nuts, eggs, cheese, grains, and other foods.

Special Diets

The Southern Mediterranean diet

The Southern Mediterranean diet is high is fresh fruits and vegetables, olive oil, garlic, tomatoes, red wine, and fish. Red meat is seldom included. Dairy intake is also limited. Fish is included two or three times a week and should not be fried or burned during cooking. Nuts and herbs and cruciferous vegetables such as cabbage, broccoli and cauliflower are regularly included in this form of diet. In a 2013 study published online in the June 2013 "JAMA Internal Medicine" journal,[15] a team of researchers from the University of California, San Francisco, found that:

"A diet high in seeds, nuts, avocados, and oil-based dressing could reduce the risk of death for men with prostate cancer".

The research studied the fat intake of 4,577 men with non-metastatic prostate cancer over a 24 year period to 2010. It concluded that by replacing just 10% of their daily carbohydrates and animal fats with healthy vegetable fats, their prostate cancer mortality risk was reduced by 29%. The study, which was not a random controlled study, also suggested a 26% reduction in death from all causes, and called for further research to be undertaken on a healthy vegetable fat diet and prostate cancer.[16] Numerous research studies have been undertaken into the interaction of high vegetable fat diets and cardiovascular disease and/or prostate cancer. These studies suggest that there is increasing evidence that high animal fat and high carbohydrate intake may play a significant role in early prostate cancer formation.[17,18] Research has suggested that the increased use of dietary micronutrients and antioxidants such as vitamins D and E, lycopene, selenium, zinc, isoflavonoids, and phytoestrogens (soy products and green tea) may offer therapeutic benefits against prostate cancer formation and subsequently to any existing prostate cancer.

Dr Myers' Diet

Dr Charles "Snuffy" Myers is well known internationally as a prostate cancer specialist who has treated men from all corners of the globe. His great success has been delivered by adherence to his three key tenets: Extensive Research, Cutting Edge Assessment and Personalised Care. He is of the view that nutrition and lifestyle are vital components in the prevention and treatment of prostate cancer. This belief has seen him recently introduce an improved and updated edition of his earlier successful book "Eating your Way to Better Health" which has been re-named *"The New Prostate Cancer Nutrition Book"*. To quote from his web site accessible via Appendix 3.

"Using indisputable research on the health-benefits of the Mediterranean Diet, this new edition tackles the most pertinent issues in the field today with evidence-based analysis".

Perhaps, an observation of interest is that the cover of his book shows the following: Avocado, tomato, onion, broccoli, beans, pomegranate, cherry, Kiwi fruit, garlic cloves and various nuts.

The Japanese Diet

Prostate cancer in Japanese men is at a significantly lower level than in those with a Western diet.[19,20] Their diet is high in fish, soy and vegetables. It is low in calories (meat) and fat. Green tea is also an important component of most meals.

Other General Dietary Comments

Pomegranate juice was found in a 2006 UCLA research study to slow or even reverse the recurrent cancer rise in PSA after initial treatment. The men's overall PSA doubling time was nearly four times slower after they drank a glass of pomegranate juice (8 fluid ounces. or 250ml) every day for 33 months. Sixteen of the 46 patients had a decrease in PSA levels. In four participants their PSA levels dropped by half.[21] The US National Cancer Institute's web site covers the issue of pomegranate juice extensively. Access it via Appendix 3.

The following are considered bad for prostate cancer (pre and post diagnosis):

Red meat and high fat dairy products

Trans fatty acids such as margarines, baked and fried food

High calcium foods such as cheeses, custard and ice creams

Pickled, salted and preserved foods

Flaxseed oil

High doses of zinc.

Homeopathy

Homeopathy is a system of alternative medicine that involves treating the patient with highly diluted substances that are designed to trigger the body's natural healing capabilities. The practice is based on the principle of treating "like with like". For example, the symptoms created by a high dose of a compound, might see these symptoms counteracted by administering a much weaker or highly diluted amount of the same compound. The use of homeopathic remedies or the use of supplements is happening at unprecedented levels. A 2006 study tested 5 Indian-sourced homeopathic remedies against MAT-LyLu prostate cancer cells in rats over 5 weeks. The small study concluded that the remedies had no direct cellular anti-cancer effect but appeared to significantly slow the progression of cancer and reduce cancer incidence and mortality in the target rats.[22]

In his book *"How to fight Prostate Cancer and Win"* Ron Gellatley outlined a number of homeopathic remedies that he used to successfully fight his prostate cancer. These included the making up of a remedy that he calls T4, which activates the T4 "killer" cells in the body and his homeopathic thymus that stimulates the thymus gland to release aggressor cells to then go on the attack.

Shark Cartilage, Bovine Tracheal Cartilage

A best-selling book published in 1992 titled *"Sharks Don't Get Cancer"* convinced many people that the taking of ground shark cartilage as a food supplement might "protect" them from cancer. However, it has been proven that many species of shark do get cancer and that there is no strong scientific evidence that shark cartilage is useful in treating or preventing cancer or other diseases. The proponents of the use of shark cartilage, as an anticancer agent, refer to the research that details its ability to stop or slow angiogenesis, the process of blood vessel development. Cancer cells rely on rapid blood vessel development for their survival and propagation.

Prior to the book referred to earlier being published, bovine tracheal cartilage consumption as a food supplement was higher than that of shark cartilage. Its proponents believe it to have similar angiogenesis properties to the shark cartilage. Additionally, it is thought to have immune system stimulating capabilities. Since the early 70's, at least a dozen clinical trials of cartilage as a cancer fighting agent have been concluded (or are still ongoing). Only 7 of these trials have had their results published in peer-reviewed journals.[23] Results of these clinical trials appear to be inconclusive as to the benefits provided by both types of cartilage. Clinical trials and research are ongoing.

Lactoferrin

As babies, we were all first exposed to lactoferrin immediately after birth when we started being breastfed by our mothers. It is an iron-binding protein found in the colostrum (new mother's milk). There is about seven times the quantity of lactoferrin in early mother's milk in humans (and cows) than exists later in the breast-feeding cycle. It is thought to protect the new born against bacterial infections and disease. Lactoferrin is produced in the exocrine glands of the body and is found in fluids of the eye, the nose, the intestines and elsewhere. It appears to have two immune-boosting functions. Firstly, it binds with iron in the blood to deprive any iron-hungry cancer cells of one of the substances that facilitate their growth. It also has the ability to release iron when necessary which makes it an excellent anti-oxidant. It is able to mop up free radicals that are coursing through our bodies at any one time. Free radicals are thought to be responsible for, or a catalyst in, the ageing process and diseases like arthritis and cancer.

Research has also identified lactoferrin as an anti-carcinogenic substance.[24] It has also been found in animal experiments, that 'iron-saturated' bovine lactoferrin is a potent natural adjuvant to augment cancer chemotherapy.[25] Lactoferrin is available, as a supplement, from health food outlets.

Summary - Complementary and Alternative Therapies

In this chapter, 18 treatments, compounds, foods, diets and mindsets are considered (referred to below collectively as 'agents'). It is fair to say that many people benefit considerably from the use of one or more of these 'agents'. Of course, some people might benefit more than others from a specific 'agent'. It is also evident that some of these 'agents' also provide benefit as regards prostate cancer. They might prevent or delay its onset; they might minimise its severity and in some cases lead to the cancer going into remission. It is not possible to summarise the impact of each of the 18 'agents' discussed in this chapter other than the one that follows:

Diets – it is clear that diet does have a significant impact on prostate cancer, both from getting the disease and limiting its progression. Followers of the Southern Mediterranean diet, in particular, have far lower incidences of prostate cancer than in men following other Western diets.

Some Factors for or against Complementary and Alternative Therapies

It is very difficult, without going into great detail, to comment further on the pros and cons of any one 'agent'. Results are often subjective and attitudes to these 'agents' and their use for prostate cancer vary considerably in the general community and across the medical profession.

Many good books are available that tell the story of complementary and alternative therapies for prostate cancer. Some have been referenced in this chapter.

Chapter 15.
The Role of Support Groups

The first line of support that you will need after being diagnosed with prostate cancer, and throughout the treatment phase, is your immediate family. It is essential to have them understand what you are going through; for them to understand your treatment regimen; and for them to be there to help you digest what you are told by your medical team. Of paramount importance is your spouse, or partner. The consequences of prostate cancer treatment, whether you are diagnosed at the local; advanced local or metastatic cancer level, are of huge concern to your wife or partner. After all, there is a reasonable likelihood that your sex life might be compromised in the short or medium term or permanently. Perhaps of even greater importance is the psychological blow that being diagnosed with a life threatening condition, might present you. Some men are able to cope with one, or both challenges very well, whilst others can just about go to pieces, and will need serious professional help to assist in regaining a positive mindset that allows them to fight the disease.

It is a battle and often it is not easy, particularly if you are diagnosed with prostate cancer at the higher risk of the scale. Your children should also be brought into the loop at an early stage. They need to understand the challenges you face and allow them the chance to participate in your recovery process. Of course, if they are under-age children, it would be far more confronting to them to know that their father has a life-threatening illness, so discretion as to what they are told is appropriate. Most couples have a circle of close friends. They too should be selectively briefed and also add themselves to the growing army of people helping you to get back to full health again, as quickly as possible. You also probably have colleagues or superiors at work who need to know that you are committed to a treatment regimen in order to restore your health. Your recovery will ensure that you continue to make an appropriate ongoing commitment to your employer's activities.

You will find that your medical team can only spend limited time with you at each stage of the diagnosis, testing and treatment phases of your condition. You cannot possibly ask all the right questions and get sufficient information from your doctors, to enable you to make the most appropriate and correct medical decision to suit your condition and your circumstances. Sure it's okay to spend hours on the internet researching options. The problem is that there is so much information out there, that it is very hard to get the right information that matches your unique position. (Author's Note: I've spent hundreds and hundreds of hours researching for this book, with the majority of information being gleaned from the Web. I have also spoken to dozens of prostate cancer survivors and many medical professionals, in addition to the dozen or so books read on the subject).

Even medical doctors, who have been diagnosed with prostate cancer, don't know which questions to ask their urologist or radiation oncologist. I played golf with a general surgeon a few months ago, who had had a radical prostatectomy six months earlier. Apparently, he had a good outcome from the surgery. However, he had almost no knowledge of the other alternative treatments available to him. He appeared vague about the two forms of brachytherapy available and had no knowledge of proton beam therapy, HIFU and other focal treatments. He did not tell me his Gleason Score, so I am unable to speculate as to whether or not he needed the treatment that he had. **(Remember I am NOT a medical doctor).** He had not considered radiation therapy either. I hypothesise that he had gone to see an urologist, who generally favoured a surgical solution to treat prostate cancer, and took the urologist's advice to have his prostate removed. Now, there is nothing wrong with his actions, other than the suggestion that he did not consider other options that might have given him an even better outcome than that achieved. Engagement with others who collectively have had a variety of treatments at a prostate cancer support group might have alerted him to other, perhaps more beneficial alternatives.

One of the issues when you question men who have had prostate cancer surgery, radiation treatment, or any other method of treating the cancer, is often too hard to pursue: **Are you impotent? Are you**

incontinent? These are extremely private questions that really cannot be asked other than by a doctor. A few men volunteer answers to these questions before being asked, as they know they are the two most vital questions, after the most important one of all, and that is, will you be free of the cancer after treatment and survive?

Many men attending prostate support groups have been through the mill and attend with a view to helping others. Others, who still have to decide on a course of treatment, attend as a learning experience. These groups often have a different modus operandi. Some meet informally over lunch; others under the auspices of a hospital or regional health centre; others are run by not-for-profit organisations like Cancer Councils; etc. It is best to access the Internet to find which groups are active in your area and how you might find out more information about attending, etc.

I recently bought a copy of Dr Jay Cohen's book *"Breakthroughs in Prostate Cancer 2014"*. It is an excellent book written by a medical doctor who practices medicine outside the genitourinary field. He was diagnosed with prostate cancer in 2011 and was booked in for surgery after a process that appeared to be very similar to that of the general surgeon that I referred to earlier. He was sent to see a nurse specialist who provided him with information about the standard treatment options. She answered his many questions, as well as suggesting he might want to investigate a local independent support group called the **"Informed Prostate Cancer Support Group" (IPCSG)**. This group meets monthly on a Saturday, a day that prevented Dr Cohen attending, due to his work commitments. However, a few of their members meet informally for lunch each week. The attendees use the lunch to update their colleagues on their status, treatment outcomes, etc. They also discuss new information that they might have gleamed from news reports, medical literature or from the Web. Dr Cohen "discovered" **DCE-MRI** and **Colour Doppler Ultrasound** at one of these lunches. His doctor had not mentioned either of these important tools in the diagnosis of prostate cancer, to him. He also became aware that the IPCSG offers more than 30 DVDs prepared from their monthly meeting lecturer's presentations. He became a regular attendee at these luncheons. In short, his attendance at the lunches convinced him to have a Colour Doppler Ultrasound and a DCE-MRI as a follow-up. The results from these two tests convinced him to join the *"Active Surveillance"* brigade. The IPCSG has a very interesting web site with a host of information and links to other pertinent prostate cancer diagnoses and treatment. It also lists details of the DVD's that are for sale at $10.00 each. Access their web site via Appendix 3.

An international prostate cancer support group, called **Us TOO International, Inc.**, exists that has 325 chapters worldwide. A significant number of these exist in the USA. Support groups are listed in 13 countries as follows:

USA (about 300); India (1); Belgium (1); The Netherlands (1); Nigeria (1); Spain (1); Australia (3); Tanzania (1); Bahamas (3); South Africa (1); Canada (7); Scotland (2); England (7).

The number in brackets indicates the number of groups in that country. Access the web site via Appendix 3. Us Too International have been operating for 24 years and have the following mission statement:

"The mission of Us TOO is to help men and their families make informed decisions about prostate cancer detection and treatment through support, education and advocacy".

I did NOT attend a structured support group, but rather called on the experiences of four or five close friends and my older brother, all of whom had faced prostate cancer before my diagnosis. Two reasons contributed to me not joining a formal group. Perhaps the most important reason was my personality. As a bit of a loner, I like researching and discovering things myself. After a 45 year career in the commercial side of science and medicine, I am well-versed in investigative research and understanding technical and medical jargon. A lesser reason for not attending a support group, was geographical, as I live 60 miles (100kms) from Sydney, Australia. Trips to the city require a 90 minutes road trip or a 30 minute drive to the nearest rail link followed by an 80 minute train trip.

However, in September 2014, I discovered that the Prostate Cancer Foundation of Australia have grown their number of support groups to 165, with one group meeting about 25 kilometres from my home. I was pleased to attend my first support group meeting recently. A local urologist was the guest speaker and the meeting was attended by about 30 men, some with spouses, and a small number of area health continence nurses and a social worker. I have resolved to attend regularly.

A number of the Proton Beam centres support an independent alumni of past prostate cancer patients. The most well-known of these is *"The Brotherhood of the Balloon"* (called BOB for short) run by Robert Marckini. It has some 7000 prostate cancer patients previously treated at the Proton Beam Therapy Centre at the Loma Linda University Medical Centre who receive a regular newsletter, reunions and other benefits.[1] Robert has also authored an excellent book on prostate cancer titled **"YOU CAN BEAT Prostate Cancer and You Don't Need Surgery to Do It"**. It is a very informative and inspiring read.

So don't forget to consider joining a prostate cancer support group.

PART 3: MY PROSTATE CANCER JOURNEY

Chapter 16.

My Prostate Cancer: Ongoing Research

In Part 1 of this book, I gave details of being diagnosed with prostate cancer and details of my follow up visit to Dr P., my first urologist. He had indicated that I was an excellent candidate for a radical prostatectomy. Using the Da Vinci® keyhole surgery system, I would have a short hospital stay and be back on the golf course in no time. However, whilst all surgical care would be taken to spare the nerve bundles that control erections, there could be no guarantee that I would maintain my ability to have an erection. Also, there was a possibility that I would also suffer from incontinence, particularly stress incontinence (the release of urine upon coughing). In fact, the chance of me having erectile dysfunction was rated at 24 to 29% with the figure for incontinence being around 30% at 6 months after surgery. Dr P advised that if I did suffer from erectile dysfunction after the operation, it was possible that my ability to have an erection might partially or wholly return over time. It might be assisted by taking Viagra, Levitra or Cialis before intercourse.

By the way, I should regress somewhat. During the consultation when I was told that I had prostate cancer, my urologist made a small drawing of my prostate and indicated where the cancerous tissue appeared in the prostate. It was present in both lobes with the left lobe containing a sizeable tumour. Nine of the 24 biopsy samples contained cancer cells. The reason I had so many samples was that I have permanent arrhythmia of the heart and take warfarin to thin the blood to lessen the risk of a stroke. I had to go on Clexane® injection treatment for the five days I was off warfarin. The larger than normal number of cores taken, would obviate the need for a medium term follow up biopsy. I was pretty disappointed that there was no computer-generated image to show the size and distribution of the tumours. However, just being told I had cancer, didn't get me going on this point. Also, there was no discussion about the option of active surveillance, probably because I had an intermediate risk cancer with a Gleason Score of 7 (3 + 4 which is far better than 4+3 as explained earlier in this book).

All of this was enough to put me right off the prospect of surgery. I have a couple of friends who I meet with once or twice a month in Sydney to discuss stocks and shares. John had had proton beam therapy in the USA some ten years or so ago. Paul had had a radical prostatectomy performed by one of Australia's leading urological surgeons about four years ago when he was 60 years of age. Whilst John and I had met Paul before his surgery, Paul was really a casual acquaintance, with us bumping into each other at investment presentations, conferences, etc. from time to time. He was unaware of proton beam therapy leading up to his surgery, nor was he made aware of it as a possible treatment by his urologist. He didn't get much input from his specialist about other forms of treatment either. He was given two choices: a radical prostatectomy or a course of external beam radiation therapy.

The various other radiation techniques such as low dose or high dose brachytherapy or HIFU, were not mentioned to him as options. When first diagnosed, Paul had a PSA of 12.5; with a Gleason Score of 7 (3+4) and his cancer was considered a Type 1c. He was unclear as to the number of biopsy cores taken and the number that contained cancerous tissue. Two thoughts come to mind, regarding Paul's decision to have surgery and his lack of understanding of his diagnosis and the various options that were open to him: firstly he had cancer and wanted to do whatever it took to rid himself as soon as possible of the scourge that is cancer and secondly, his medical team did not appear to share with him vital information that they should have, so as to give him real choice as to the alternative therapies open to him. In my view, this was not a good situation to have to face at a time of acute anxiety. Well, what was the outcome of the surgery? He had a complete inability to have an erection and incontinence to the point where he has to wear a urinary pad all the time.

My friend 'Michael', who I caught up with at my school reunion in South Africa, also had erectile dysfunction after surgery and even with pharmaceutical assistance, found sex a chore only to be endured for the benefit of his wife.

Side Effects of Current Treatments

% of Patients Treated

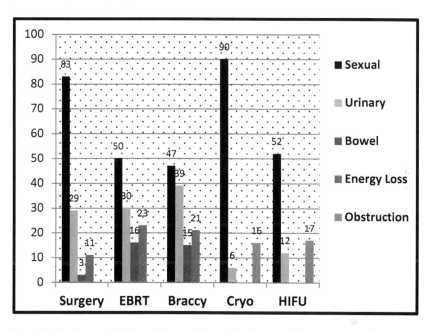

Graph: Courtesy of LaZure Scientific Inc. developers of LDAC technology

In my research into the treatment options I faced, I came across a book titled *"Surviving Cancer with Proton Therapy: Road to Nami Island"*, written by York L. Phillips and Curtis Poling. The central character in the book called "Joe" undergoes successful proton beam therapy in Korea. However, in the lead up to deciding on this treatment, he visited a number of leading physicians each of whom recommended his speciality as being the most appropriate for Joe, considering his PSA, Gleason Score, etc. Now, all could be correct in their claim, but some treatment types might have been better than others. (Author's Note: "Joe" is a fictional figure, but the story line is based on fact). My wife tells me that I am often cynical. She is probably right as I saw the above example manifested by some of the medical specialists I encountered, whilst researching my treatment options and indeed in the preparation of this book.

Back to Paul. He became aware of proton beam therapy when John and I were discussing it in his presence (This was during the period I was researching my treatment options). Paul was interested to learn more about John's treatment at Loma Linda in the USA. Of course, he found out too late of the benefits available to men having treatments other than a radical prostatectomy. His interest and geno-urinary condition had quite an impact on me. It convinced me to do something as a layman (and a prostate cancer sufferer), to spread the word on the options that are available to newly-diagnosed men and to keep track of technical and medical developments in the field.

At my second post diagnosis meeting with my urologist, he asked how my consideration of the various treatment options was progressing. I was able to tell him that I definitely would not consider a radical prostatectomy, due to the unacceptably high incidence of erectile dysfunction and incontinence. He was a little disappointed that I hadn't followed his advice, but he recognised my right to make this decision. I also told him that I wasn't too keen on external beam radiation therapy (or its newer forms) either. The main reason I advanced were:

The high prospect of loss of erectile function

The high incontinence risk

An inability to have further radiation should cancer return down the track

The slight possibility of secondary cancers forming as a result of the radiation dose received.

My research at this stage had focussed on two treatment formats: Proton beam therapy and HIFU. My urologist was somewhat familiar with proton beam therapy, which he suggested was still considered an experimental technique. (Some 100,000 men over 30 years had undergone PBT by this time!! – How long do they need to realise it's a main stream cancer-killing tool?). He also suggested that it was likely to be very expensive, would not be covered under Australian Medicare insurance scheme or by my private health fund, as it was only available in America. (In fact, there were/are about 15 proton beam centres around the world that accept foreigners and are able to converse with you in English)!

Chapter 17.
Was HIFU the Answer?

My second technique of interest was High Frequency Ultrasound (HIFU) in which an ultrasonic probe is inserted in the rectum and the whole prostate gland is ablated (under precise computer control) by the ultrasonic energy. The system heats the prostate tissue to more than 70°C (158°F), thus killing the prostate and cancer tissue.

My interest in this procedure was because the treatment was quick and simple (a one-off 3 hour procedure), with a likelihood of fewer and less severe side effects. A search of the internet had indicated that about 6 urologists in Sydney used the technique. I also found a news release from one of the two HIFU instrument manufacturers congratulating one of Australia's most well-known and proficient cancer urologists for undergoing overseas training on their system a year earlier. He had begun to treat patients locally with their HIFU system. I happened to be acquainted with one of the doctors who used HIFU (from a previous golf match). Dr L practised at a prestigious cancer institute and was highly regarded in his area of speciality. A referral was obtained and a few weeks later I found myself running down the road from the station to get to my appointment on time after a late arriving train had intervened. Fortunately, the doctor was running 15 minutes late so I had time to cool down and feel like a proper person again before I saw the doctor.

Dr L examined my medical record and pathology report and did the regular digital rectal examination. No lumpiness was found during the DRE. We discussed HIFU. He advised that he still uses the technique but only sparingly, particularly in men in the late seventies and eighties. He was of the view that whole prostate gland ablation was too radical a solution in my case considering the size and distribution of the tumours in my prostate. (My tumours were all adenocarcinomas which are the most common prostate cancer tumour type). He suggested that high dose brachytherapy might be a more beneficial approach to take considering my age, physical fitness, pathology, etc. I suggested to him that my sample of one person (my brother) undergoing this type of treatment had shown a recurrence of the cancer eight years later. His response was that there is always a small percentage of patients who have recurrences, even after radical prostatectomies, or other forms of treatment. All it needs is for a few cancer cells to survive the treatment, and then to re-establish themselves as a threatening tumour over time. He suggested that he could refer me to a good radiation oncologist based at the hospital adjacent to his institute to arrange the HDR brachytherapy. This I declined, as I would prefer a radiation oncologist who practised much nearer to my home as after the HDR brachytherapy treatment, I would need to undergo about 30 doses of x-ray radiation over about six weeks. This assumed that I would decide on HDR brachytherapy, which was a decision not yet made.

At about this time, which was six weeks or so after my second post diagnosis visit, I had reason to contact the private clinic that was named as now doing HIFU, only to discover that they were "no longer using HIFU". No explanation was forthcoming. I understand that at least two of the other doctors doing the HIFU treatment in Sydney rent the device from the manufacturer (a different brand from the private clinic above) for the procedure. The cost of the procedure was about A$14,000 of which about 75% would be funded by Medicare and my own private health insurance fund. The private hospital fees for set up time, theatre time and recovery would be an additional A$4,000, which would be fully met by my private health insurance, except for a small payment of A$250.

Chapter 18.
A Third Urologist enters the Picture

I discussed my next possible move with my wife, who had years of experience as a scrub nurse working with the best surgeons and urologists at Sydney's leading private hospital. She named two specialists who both had HIFU experience at the hospital and were at the top of their profession. She suggested that I get my general practitioner to refer me to one of these two men. Lo and behold! One of them had the same names as my schoolboy professional cricket coach. The coach, who had spent twenty years as a top leg-spin bowler playing County cricket in England, was a huge man who had fingers like bananas. In fact, he was the only man I have seen who could hold three cricket balls (the size of large apples) upside down in one hand! When he ran in to bowl (a type of pitch!), the ball was completely invisible due to the size of his hand. Guess which specialist I chose? The cricket coach's namesake. A referral was obtained and the appointment arranged.

I was in for another shock. When ushered into his consulting room, I was surprised to find Dr T to be a smallish man, just the opposite in size to my former cricket coach. However, I took to him immediately, due to his quiet, but confident manner, and his ability to impart quality medical information in a straightforward and fully understandable way. After reviewing my pathology records, hearing of my interest in HIFU and PBT, and asking me numerous questions about my urinary flow etc., he suggested the following course of action:

He concurred with Dr L's view that I might do better than HIFU, by having High Dose Brachytherapy followed by x-ray radiation.

He wanted to do a urine flow test to determine how completely I emptied my bladder.

Dependent on the results of the flow test, he might undertake a transurethral resection of the prostate (TURP) to improve prostate flow before the radiation treatment might begin.

After a three months healing time after the TURP procedure, I would be ready for the HDR brachytherapy and subsequent x-ray radiation.

The urine flow test was scheduled for the following week and I reported to the hospital after drinking the requisite amount of water before arriving. The test equipment measures the volume of urine released from the body, the speed of its release and the length of time it takes for its release. It is very simple test requiring you to urinate into a large funnel that collects the urine in a flask that is on a weighing scale. It sends this data to a computer which prints out a report. The test, called an uroflowmetry test, is over in a few minutes. Dr T was able to advise me that my flow was below par and as such I should undergo the TURP procedure as soon as it could be arranged. A fortnight later, I returned to the hospital to have the TURP operation. It was certainly a more involved procedure than the simple uroflowmetry test.

The TURP procedure calls for removal of tissue from the prostate to improve the urine flow. It can also be used in some elderly or frail men to remove (large) parts of the prostate instead of undergoing a more demanding radical prostatectomy. The procedure calls for the insertion of an instrument called a resectoscope though the penis and urethra into the prostate. The instrument is about 12 inches (30cm) long and one-half inch (13mm) in diameter. It contains valves that control irrigating fluid, a light and an electrical loop that cuts tissue and seals blood vessels. The wire loop is guided by the surgeon so it can remove the obstructing tissue one piece at a time. The pieces of tissue are carried by fluid into the bladder and flushed out at the end of the procedure.

The procedure is colloquially referred to as 'having a re-bore'. The literature reports that a number of side effects could follow the re-bore: - these include bleeding after the operation and retrograde ejaculation – most men are able to have erections and orgasms after the surgery. However, they may not ejaculate, because the bladder neck is removed along with prostatic tissue. This causes the ejaculate to collect with urine and pass out in the next urination.

In my case, the procedure was green laser-based and somewhat different to the above. The tissue, that was slowing the flow of my urine, was burned away by the laser. This resulted in far less bleeding and is well suited to people, like myself, who are on anti-coagulation therapy. A side effect that I experienced was a need to go to the toilet urgently and frequently to urinate. As the weeks passed, this condition became less and less of a problem. There was also a little blood in my urine for some days after the procedure.

A follow up visit was made to Dr T some weeks later to check my progress after the TURP and to firm up a visit to his recommended radiation oncologist, a Dr W. However, I still had not fully accepted that I would follow through with his recommended treatment. I thought that I would meet Dr W. and see what he had to say. It was now mid-September 2012. I had some concern about the cancer cells in my prostate that were multiplying as every day went by and might at any time try to escape through the prostate wall into the lymph nodes and/or seminal vesicles. It was this human trait of wanting to be rid of the cancer there and then, raising its head again.

I Start Androgen Deprivation Therapy

After a discussion with Dr T, I asked the doctor to prescribe Zoladex®, which is an androgenic drug therapy (fully described in Part 2 of this book), which would keep the cancer cells starved of their food - testosterone and its more dangerous variant, dihydrotestosterone. Zoladex® comes in the form of a syringe that sees the Zoladex® injected below the skin of the abdomen, where it leeches into the bloodstream over three months. As my wife, Pam, opened the package, I noted the needle to be very sizeable. In fact, I had never seen a bigger one for use with humans! I asked her to do the injection and she agreed. I further, asked her to carefully read the instructions on how to operate the syringe, as it had a complicated-looking blue safety device on it. I lay down on the bed with my belly exposed and Pam with the needle poised. After the necessary sterilisation of the injection zone with a sterilizing agent, in went the needle. Then the fumbling started. She could not get the safety device released, so that the syringe contents could be emptied into my torso. Eventually, I had to hold the syringe whose needle was more than an inch into my body so that she could collect the instructions that were on the table 15 feet or so away. After a quick read, the safety device was released and the Zoladex® started flowing into my system. A rather funny, but painful experience. I made sure that the next injection which was due in mid-January 2012 would be less painful and less hilarious.

Chapter 19.

Proton Beam Therapy Re-Visited

I had established that it was possible to have proton beam therapy at two centres, Loma Linda University Medical Centre (LLUMC) outside Los Angeles, USA or the National Cancer Centre (NCC) in Seoul, South Korea. My friend John had fully acquainted me with his Loma Linda experience and I had received a package of information from KMI International Inc. KMI facilitate matters for international patients wanting to attend treatment at the proton beam centre at the NCC in Seoul. I thought that I would request quotations from both hospitals and complete application forms. This included making copies of my histology reports from the pathologists as well as providing each centre with the 'negatives' of my bone scan and CT scan, which showed no signs of prostate cancer being metastasised outside of the prostate gland. Both proton beam centres only treat prostate cancer patients with localised cancer (confined to the prostate gland itself).

The quotation came in from Loma Linda. It was US$85,000 for treatment only. Accommodation could be arranged by them close to the centre, but would be for my account. Due to it being in a semi-rural setting a hire car would be needed for the nine week stay (39 treatment days, plus three days for the initial testing, set up, treatment plan development, etc.). Of course, I would want my wife, Pam, to accompany me so overall I was looking at no change out of US$100,000. At my friend John's insistence, I had been in contact with Bob Marckini, who runs the Brotherhood of the Balloon support group for the alumni of the proton beam centre at LLUMC. I also downloaded his book via Amazon Inc. It is called **"YOU CAN BEAT Prostate Cancer and You Don't Need Surgery to Do It"**. An excellent read and it's very informative. Bob was very generous with his time and answered numerous questions that I had about PBT and the LLUMC.

Before I had my first consultation with Dr W, I heard back from Korea. I was medically acceptable to them and if I accepted their quotation of US$56,000, they could schedule a treatment spot for me within about three weeks. Their quotation included 39 treatment sessions, a three day session of initial tests, set up and treatment planning, accommodation in a two-bedroomed luxury apartment in downtown Seoul, a driver to take us to and from the hospital each day, a cell phone (with 300 hours of free air time) to contact their English-speaking concierge in the case of need, and a free continental breakfast each week day. All we had to pay for was the air travel, other meals, food and the cost of sightseeing. The two questions were, did I really need PBT and where the Koreans the ones to deliver it?

Chapter 20.
Enter the Radiation Oncologist

It was time to see Dr W, the radiation oncologist. At least I knew before seeing him that I had one option approved and that was PBT at the NCC in Korea. Dr W was very thorough. He explained that I would have about 20 hollow tubes inserted via a template into my prostate via the perineum area. Radioactive-tipped needles would then be introduced via the hollow tubes into the prostate. These would be left in place for some minutes (can't recall the exact time), then withdrawn and automatically placed in a lead-lined storage safe. The template and hollow tubes would remain in situ over-night (a very uncomfortable night I'm told). The next morning, the needles are re-inserted and remain in situ for a similar time period, before the procedure is completed.

I was to start the x-ray treatment a week after the brachytherapy procedure. Dr W uses an IMRT system which definitely limits the x-ray exposure to the healthy tissue adjacent to the prostate. In six weeks, after the delivery of 28 fractions, I would be as right as rain with my PSA expected to drop to negligible levels over the coming months. The cost of the procedure was to be A$33,000 (then US$31,350). (A$13,000 out of my pocket with the rest chargeable to my health insurance fund and Medicare). They also offered a new type of gel injection for about A$3,000 which would separate the prostate from the rectal wall, which would just about prevent any rectal radiation damage. See Chapter 7 for details of this gel. I have subsequently found out much more about this gel, called **SpaceOAR**®. It is suitable for photon and proton radiation techniques. If I had been more familiar with its benefits, I would have insisted on it being included in my radiation treatment. Dr W didn't particularly like my ongoing interest in proton beam therapy. He tried his best to convince me that the Bragg Peak Effect provided by proton radiation was not as controllable as I understood and the result that I would obtain might be sub-optimal. However, he did schedule me to undergo the HDR brachytherapy procedure for the second week in

January. (The healing process from the TURP had to be completed before radiation treatment could commence). A final reflection; the bill for almost an hour consultation was a very low A$165, which surprised me. My cynical streak is emerging again. Perhaps, the treatment cost would cover this low initial consultation fee, many times over. We will hear more from or about Dr W. soon.

Chapter 21.
Enter the Case for Hyperthermia

A few days after the October consultation with Dr W, I received a phone call from John. He told me that he had coffee with an old friend, whom he had not seen for a while, who had six months earlier returned to Sydney after having had prostate cancer treatment in Germany. He went on to tell me that his friend, Bill, had another younger family friend (Brian) who had more recently gone to the same clinic just outside Munich to have the same treatment. I had been aware that hyperthermia treatment for all types of cancer had been happening in Germany for years, and I had looked into the work being done by Dr Douwes at the Clinic St Georg at Bad Aibling, near Munich. I was also aware of the work being done by Dr med Peter Wolf at his clinic in Hannover.

I downloaded Dr Wolf's book *"Innovations in Biological Cancer Therapy"* from Amazon and carefully studied its contents and read the many research papers, which back up his various treatment protocols. Both these clinics treat prostate cancer with heat radiation and work on the premise that cancer cells are unable to survive prolonged heating to above 42° C (108° F). This is due to the tumour's poor vascular network not being able to dissipate the induced heat, as is the case with healthy tissue with their superior vascular structure. The heating of the cancer cells also leads to the release of heat shock proteins (HSP) by the cancer cells. The HSP make the cancer cells far more vulnerable to attack by both one's own immune system and low dose chemical or biological agents. Unfortunately, Bill left on a four week business trip to Thailand the day after meeting John, so I was unable to catch up with him face to face. A few emails back and forth made hyperthermia more promising to me.

A day or two later, I received an email from LLUMC saying *"Congratulations. You have been accepted to undergo proton beam therapy with us. A time slot is expected to be available in forty-five days"* (early January 2013). Gee – I now had two options from which to choose. I went back to LLUMC and ask for a listing of Australians and New Zealanders that had PBT at Loma Linda and who would be willing to give me feedback on their experience. The list that duly arrived by email was much longer than I expected and I made email contact with a few people who lived in Sydney or its surroundings. Every reply was very positive and endorsed what John had told me previously.

At this time, I also emailed KMI for details of any Australians or New Zealanders who had PBT at the NCC. I received contact details for an Australian, called John, and a New Zealander called Derek, who had sold his house and downsized to help pay for his treatment in Korea. Both have testimonials on the www.protonkorea.com web site. I made email contact with John, who lives almost 1500 miles north of my home, which prevented a face-to-face meeting. He was very generous in answering my many questions, both about the treatment and about living in Korea for 10 weeks or so. He completed his PBT treatment at the NCC in March 2012, and at the time of last contact, he was still as positive as ever about the treatment, his recovery and every other aspect of his Korean experience. It was interesting to note that John had received 28 radiation treatments, rather than the standard 39 sessions offered to all international prostate cancer patients at the NCC. This called for the delivery of a slightly higher daily radiation dose to compensate for the fewer treatments.

After a bit of too and froing, I obtained the email address of Brian, who had undertaken a course of hyperthermia at the Clinic St Georg in Germany. After a few emails, at last, I had an opportunity to speak with him over the phone. This lengthy discussion suggested to me that hyperthermia was a really viable option for me. Brian had had his treatment some 6 months previously (not long after Bill's treatment). His treatment program was as follows:

Thursday afternoon - Arrive at clinic and have general examination and blood tests

Friday - Undergo the three hour transurethral treatment followed by being placed on a drip

Saturday morning - A further drip during the morning. (Left clinic until Monday am)

Monday - Second three hour treatment

Tuesday - further drip

Wednesday - discharged at noon.

His treatment involved a probe being inserted via the urethra into the region of the prostate. This probe was activated by radiofrequency energy to heat the prostatic tissue to 47 – 48° C (117° F) with the temperature being closely monitored by a temperature sensor built into the probe. The procedure was done under local anaesthetic and was painless. The drips he had, included a series of chemical and biological agents designed to stimulate his immune system to attack the heat shock proteins that had "put their hands up" after being subjected to the two sessions of heat. A six months course of Androgen Deprivation Therapy was also commenced on his arrival for treatment.

The clinic found it possible to offer him a somewhat Spartan room "in house" for the duration of his treatment. The total cost of the treatment was around A$10,000 (US$8,000 today). His input, together with the research data presented to me by the clinic convinced me that hyperthermia was a cost effective solution to my prostate cancer problem. It appeared to have fewer side-effects than almost all other treatments. One of their research papers[1] reported:

Patients at the earliest stage of prostate cancer, (stages Type I, NO, MO) 16 men out of 16 (100%) had complete remission. At five years post treatment, all of the 14 surviving men were still in complete remission. The two that had died in the interim, died from conditions other than cancer. Patients with early stage disease, (T2 a-b, NO, MO) 32 men out of 32 (100%), also had complete remissions. The size of the study was small, but obtaining 100% complete remission at 5 years can't be ignored.

There were three other questions regarding hyperthermia that I needed answered. Firstly, the Israel-made machine, used by the clinic, appeared to be out of production, with no apparent replacement available. Secondly, the transurethral hyperthermia (TUH) treatment appeared to be only available in Germany and Austria. Whole body hyperthermia clinics exist in many countries, including Australia. If the TUH treatment was so good, why had it not been adopted elsewhere? Thirdly, the US FDA had approved the use of microwave hyperthermia more than ten years ago, but only when it was followed by radiation therapy. Why was radio frequency induced-heating not considered for approval? I intended to find answers to these questions before making a final commitment to attend the Clinic St Georg.

The clinic asked me to forward my prostate cancer medical records to them for their review. A few days later I was disappointed to receive an email from them which stated: *"Regrettably, we are NOT able to accept you as a patient due to the fact that you have had a TURP operation, and the resultant scar tissue is not compatible with our treatment regime"*. I had pretty well concluded that transurethral RF hyperthermia was the way to rid myself of my prostate cancer. Subject to satisfactory answers to the three questions posed above, I was "almost on the plane" to a part of the world that I know well and very much like. (In the last month of my working career seven years ago, I led an Australian Trade Delegation to Munich, Darmstadt and Frankfurt. We spent a week staying in a village near Bad Ailing and very much enjoyed the hotel there. Visiting the Max Plank Institute, the Fraunhofer Institute and other world class research centres in Munich on the business trip was also a great experience. The hotel had to rush in new supplies of our favourite red wine, Robert Mondavi Cabernet Sauvignon (Californian Napa Valley) from their suppliers!

As I still had not given up hope for a hyperthermia solution, I contacted Dr med Peter Wolf's clinic in Hannover, pointing out that I had been rejected for transurethral RF hyperthermia treatment by the Clinic St Georg. The Dr Wolf clinic confirmed that the scar tissue problem would not allow them to do the transurethral RF hyperthermia treatment either. They were of the view that they could still assist me in my fight against the cancer.

They proposed the following alternative treatment program:

"You will receive daily 2 hours local-regional hyperthermia and once per week whole body hyperthermia, which takes about 3.5 hours. During these treatments you will receive the individually prescribed

intravenous infusions, and you will orally take daily the additionally prescribed medication". The cost of the three week treatment as an out-patient at the clinic was to be Euro 3,500 per week, plus Euro 1,500 to 2,000 for pharmaceuticals during the treatment and for three months' supply for use after the clinic visit.

Their quotation also included the following:

"Due to our many years of therapeutic experience, we have come to believe that only a combination of orthodox medicine and the broad spectrum of the alternative medicine, the way we apply it, offers promising ways in cancer therapy. This opinion is shared by a growing number of university experts in cancer therapy. Today, they also see the necessity for personalised and individual treatment with medication and food supplements. It is important, that the chosen therapies and their respective aims are complementary in order to increase the success of the overall therapy. This is the reason why our complementary therapeutic offer is in line with traditional methods and creates a receptive and supportive environment.

Our therapy methods are designed to work on different levels:

Destroying tumour cells

Strengthening the immune system

Stabilisation of the detoxification processes of the metabolism

Optimisation of the anabolism

Increasing the quality of life

Creating a supportive environment in handling the disease."

After reading Dr Wolf's book referred to earlier, I felt that his approach to cancer treatment was likely to lead to a good outcome. However, I was interested in having transurethral hyperthermia, as Dr Douwes from the Clinic St. Georg had reported, that offered me an almost certain prospect of 100% cancer remission (admittedly based on a small study sample size). So regretfully, other hyperthermia treatments were not for me.

A little more detail on Brian's prostate cancer history before he had the hyperthermia experience: He was 51 when his PSA jumped from

4.2 to 4.7 over the period of a year. His urologist suggested a biopsy, which was subsequently done. None of the 10 cores showed cancer. He missed a PSA test the following year probably due to complacency after he had received the "all clear" after the biopsy. At 53, he had another PSA test done and he was shocked to see his PSA result come in at 7.0. This time his urologist undertook a 25 core biopsy which sure enough found cancer. It was a Gleason 7 (3+4). His urologist suggested a radical prostatectomy and he was booked in to have the surgery.

Whilst he was waiting for the operation with some fear, dread and specific concerns about the threat of incontinence and erectile dysfunction, he received an email from a fellow prostate cancer sufferer, who suggested he check out hyperthermia at the Clinic St. Georg in Germany. Unfortunately, he put the email aside, without fully researching it at that time. Apparently, he decided to undertake a herbal-based treatment that had shown promising signs in a USA university study. After a few months he abandoned this treatment, when his PSA continued to increase. When it reached 14, he again elected to have the radical prostatectomy. Whilst he was awaiting the operation and still harbouring concerns about the possible side effects, he again "found" the email about the Clinic St. Georg. A few days of concentrated research resulted in him again cancelling his surgery and electing to have the transurethral hyperthermia treatment done in Germany.

On his return to Australia in February 2012, Brian had two 3D Power Doppler Ultrasounds done over a period of a few months. They showed the prostate had shrunk by 25%, and confirmed that the prostate was effectively dead with no sign of the tell-tale cancerous vascularity remaining. It did detect a number of prostatic stones that had formed from prostatic gland secretions into pearl-like calcified deposits. These stones were unlikely to be problematic.

Chapter 22.
How Do You Get to a Final Treatment Choice?

I was scheduled to have a Prostate Ultrasound Volume Study at the radiation oncologist's rooms in Sydney, in preparation for the high dose brachytherapy treatment due to be done in January 2013. The Study was to be done on the 27th November. It was getting down to the wire as to me possibly having brachytherapy. It was time to make a decision: HDR brachytherapy or Proton Beam Therapy. I had discarded other treatment types.

It would have been helpful if I had a worksheet or check list that I could go through to try to help me decide. Whilst researching material for this book, I came across such a worksheet designed by Dr John McHugh, an urologist and prostate cancer sufferer, from Georgia, USA. He is also the author of a best-selling book on prostate cancer called *"The Decision: Your prostate biopsy shows cancer. Now what?"* He also has a very extensive web site, a regular newsletter and a blog on prostate cancer. Access his web site via Appendix 3. His worksheet did not exactly contain all the questions that I would find appropriate to my HDR brachytherapy versus proton beam therapy conundrum and, at the time I had to make this decision, I was not aware of Dr McHugh or his worksheet.

The issue became one of trying to weigh up the likely side effects and possible recurrence of the cancer after each form of treatment. My research led me to believe that proton beam therapy offered the best outcome on both, fewer side effects and less likelihood of a recurrence. I must say, that at the time I made the decision, I was not thinking with absolute clarity as I was still under the "let's get rid of the cancer now" syndrome. However, the decision to go with the vastly more costly PBT had been made and I now had to make a decision between going to Loma Linda in the USA or to the NCC in Seoul, Korea.

My research into the NCC revealed it was regarded as one of the most advanced cancer treatment centres in the world. It was equipped with the very latest technology and the IBA brand PBT system and its cyclotron were relatively new. So there were no concerns from a technical stand point. The people at KMI were very easy to deal with. I should explain that Curtis Poling, who runs KMI and his daughter Andrea Poling, are based in the USA. Curtis had previously been treated at Loma Linda for prostate cancer. Emails to Andrea were answered very promptly and contained all the material or answers requested. Email discussion with John from Central Queensland, as a past patient at the National Cancer Centre, was also very supportive of a Korean solution.

I came across a fellow Australian who previously had prostate cancer treatment at one of the regional proton beam centres in Japan. He had hired a translator to work with the non-English-speaking medical staff at the facility. Whilst, he achieved a good outcome, he would not go through that again, purely due to the language barrier.

It was clear that language would not be a significant problem at the NCC as the head of their proton beam facility, Dr Cho Kwan-Ho, had spent 13 years practicing in the USA. Most of his medical colleagues responsible for treating other types of cancer were also trained in the USA. KMI's presence in Seoul is via Wendy Lee, who is a charming (and attractive) young lady who had done under-graduate studies in Australia. She acted as a concierge, meeting international patients at the airport, introducing them to the NCC staff, arranging the daily driver, taking them to the superb apartment complex (DMC Ville) and to the local supermarket located in the World Cup 2008 stadium about a mile from the DMC Ville in the centre of high tech Digital Media City. A local cell phone to contact Wendy or anyone else was also included in the package. All this would cost US$55,900. With the then favourable US$ to A$ rate of exchange, the all up cost, including economy airfares for the 10 hour flight, was going to be around A$55,000.

The LLUMC quote was for up to 45 treatment sessions and including medical costs only, came in at US$85,000. With air fares to LA and back, a hire car and accommodation costs added we would see no change from US$100,000 (then A$95,000). Whilst I had every confidence that the Loma Linda treatment and support plan was the best available anywhere, the extra A$40,000 had to come out of our pockets, with no possible re-imbursement by our health insurance fund.

Chapter 23.

The Decision is Made: It's Proton Beam Therapy in Korea

I have travelled to the USA numerous times and have really enjoyed the country and its people. Similarly, I have visited Japan many times and have experienced Tokyo and many regional centres. I was interested in sampling the Korean culture and comparing it to that of Japan. So the die was cast: Pam and I decided that we would accept the KMI offer to have treatment at the National Cancer Centre in Seoul and made steps to arrange a date for the start of treatment. They were delighted to hear we were coming and set down the 7th January, 2013 as our first day at the NCC.

One thing that did worry us and that was the weather in winter in Korea. We live adjacent to the ocean near Sydney and have an average temperature in January/February of about 30° C (86° F) with some days getting up to 40° C (104° F). Seoul on the other hand, had January/February temperatures down to as low as minus 25° C (minus 13° F) and that's ignoring the snow, frozen footpaths, chill factor, etc. Unfortunately, as we were to travel in peak holiday season, we could not get any special deals on travel and finally booked two return economy tickets on Asiana Air, one of the two Korean-owned airlines that fly to Australia.

I had one last task to do before preparing for our Christmas season and that was to communicate with Dr W regarding my decision not to proceed with the HDR brachytherapy treatment. I tried to contact him unsuccessfully by phone over a few days, and for some reason did not leave a message. After the third or fourth attempt, I did leave a message to the effect that I would not be proceeding with my treatment with them and for them to cancel my Prostate Ultrasound Volume Study appointment. I added that I had decided to undergo proton beam therapy in Korea. I concluded the call with an apology for not following through with treatment with him and thanked him for his input up to then. A few days later, I was surprised to receive, a copy of a letter addressed to my (third) urologist (Dr T) by Dr W. He said that it was a little sad that I had been persuaded that proton treatment is more effective than brachytherapy. He went onto state that looking at proton therapy versus other external beam radiation treatments, showed that proton beam treatment was no more effective than other radiation methods, and on par with surgery. It was certainly not shown to be better than their brachytherapy program. He concluded the technical part of the letter with two statements: *"...it is a single fraction each day from one direction only and as such there are certain radiobiological issues that imply that this is a less than ideal way of delivering such treatment. .... he does unfortunately run a relatively high risk of rectal complication that he will need to have dealt with on his return."* He concluded by wishing me well.

He had every right to write this letter. However, I was a little miffed when I received it. His comment about me receiving a single daily fraction is not quite right as one gets two exposures, one through each hip per session. The newer pencil beam scanning PBT systems irradiate different parts of the prostate sequentially during one session, so his comment is clearly incorrect, when considering the very latest systems. He is considering PBT versus IMRT or RapidArc® in which multiple fractions attack the target from different directions during each session. His comment about the relatively high risk of rectal complications has some merit, as I did experience minor rectal bleeding some six months after the treatment concluded which persisted for eight months, until March this year. More details on this matter later in the book.

I called the hospital pathology department who last had my histology slides from my prostate biopsy only to be told that I couldn't have them! The NCC insisted that I bring them with me to Korea. A phone call to my first urologist saw him spring to the rescue. They were released to him and I was able to collect them and pack them carefully into my suitcase (the slides are very thin glass) Passports and visas were sorted out and we were just about ready to go.

By pure coincidence, I played golf with a Korean member of my golf club a few days before departure. He gave me a few valuable pointers as regards Seoul and Korea. One thing he said worried me somewhat: you cannot use foreign credit cards to withdraw funds from local Korean bank ATM's. I always draw foreign local currency from local banks when travelling. I have found it to be the simplest, safest and cheapest form of accessing foreign currency. I thought this to be incorrect information, but I couldn't take a chance, so the next morning I visited my bank to arrange a travel card that would definitely work in Korea. All our heavy overcoats, gloves, long thermal underwear, beanie's, etc. were aired ready for use in what promised to be a very challenging environment for us Aussies (who migrated to Australia from South Africa in 1979).

Chapter 24.
The Pre-Treatment Program in Korea

As Pam and I approached the Sydney International Airport, the mercury hit 38° C (101° F). It was the warmest day of the Australian summer. We were soon on our way on our Asiana Airlines non-stop flight to Seoul. The service on board was exemplary, as you would expect from an airline that had been voted the best international carrier a year earlier. Just prior to landing, the captain came on over the intercom and said it was a very cold evening in Seoul – in fact it was minus 20° C (minus 4° F). Snow and ice were everywhere.

A quick passage through customs and immigration saw us met by the KMI concierge, Wendy Lee and the driver, Mr Chow. We were soon on a snow-covered highway speeding towards our accommodation at the DMC Ville apartments some 45 kilometres away and just 8 kilometres from the Seoul City Hall. We were soon settled into our two bedroomed, two bath-roomed luxury apartment that was to be our home for the next nine weeks or so. Wendy said she would meet us at 10am the next morning (Monday) to take us to the nearby giant HomePlus supermarket under the World Cup Stadium to buy food and groceries. We completed our continental breakfast in the breakfast room of the complex, which is only available to international visitors to Korea, before Wendy collected us for our first Korean shopping experience. HomePlus was huge and of course everything was in Korean. An hour later, we went through the checkout with a full trolley and were presently surprised at the value received. It was perhaps two-third of Australian prices or even less. Wendy dropped us off at the apartment and said she would return at 9.00am the next morning to take us to the NCC which was 25 kilometres away towards the North Korean border. The centre of Seoul is 55 kilometre from the Demilitarized Zone between North and South Korea. We spent the rest of the day settling in and exploring the 200 apartment complex. Its facilities include an indoor golf driving range, a putt-putt course, a 25 m heated under cover swimming pool, squash courts, children's play room and a very large, fully-equipped gym with an English-speaking instructor. As a keen golfer, I thought that I would be able to work on my golf swing whilst I was in residence!

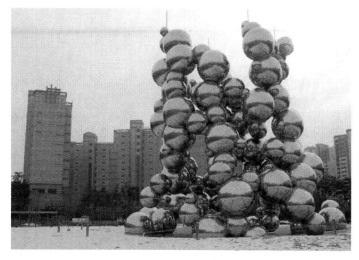

Image: Our Luxury Apartment Complex left back; Millennium Park in foreground.

At 9.00am sharp, Wendy and Mr Chow met us in the foyer, where we were joined by Jan, Henry and Henry's wife, Helen. Henry was into his 7th week of treatment whereas Jan was, like me, about to start treatment. Wendy drove Jan, Pam and I to the National Cancer Centre, with Mr Chow driving Henry and Helen there via a very icy and snow-covered freeway. The 30 minute trip was completed without incident and we arrived at the National Cancer Centre. It was a huge multi-storey hospital that looked ultra-smart and modern. We parked in the underground car park adjacent to the Proton Beam Centre and went into the equally impressive Centre to start a day of briefings, and various tests. As we entered the Centre, I noticed a large picture of the NCC with the caption below it stating:

"THE BEST CANCER TREATMENT CENTRE IN THE WORLD".

I thought to myself, that's very comforting.

After completing various forms and handing over my biopsy slides, and CT scan negatives, I had my weight and blood pressure checked. My blood pressure was higher than normal, perhaps due to underlying sub-conscious anxiety, as I was about to start treatment. I was given an injection of a radioactive tracer, to prepare me for my afternoon bone scan. Also a blood sample was taken to check my PSA and testosterone levels. Earlier, we had noticed a noticeboard at the control room level of the PBT Centre that contained the photos of international patients that had recently completed PBT treatment at the facility. The photo of John from Central Queensland and his wife was included. Also included was a photo of an eight year old girl with her parents. She had completed a course of 56 treatments for a brain stem tumour. I learnt later that she would almost certainly have died, if it was not for her PBT treatment.

We were ushered into a VIP private ward on the 11th floor of the hospital to await our 1.30pm appointment with Dr Cho, who was the head radiation oncologist for lung, head and neck, central nervous system, prostate cancer, stereotactic radiation and PBT at the Centre. After a while we felt a little peckish, so we went across the main road to a Paris Baguette pastry shop that we had spotted as we arrived at the NCC. We had been told about this chain of 500 shops that sell the most delicious cakes and pastries outside of Paris itself. The view from our 11th floor waiting room was towards Seoul. Whilst it was a little hazy, we could see the scope of the city of Ilsandong, one of the 15 or so satellite cities that surround Seoul. Twenty to thirty storey apartment blocks were everywhere.

Pam and I were escorted into see Dr Cho. He thanked us for selecting his facility for treatment and said we had made the right decision to have PBT as he was convinced it was very effective and carried minimal side effects. He did say that I might possibly have some rectal bleeding some six months down the track, but that it would soon pass and shouldn't cause me any further trouble in the future. He explained that at each radiation session, a balloon-like catheter would be inserted in my rectum and it would be filled with water. Its purpose was to press the prostate forwards so that it would always be in the exact same position. He also indicated that I should drink 500mL of water at least 30 minutes before each radiation session. The final question to be settled at the meeting was the number of radiation sessions I would have. I had been quoted for the standard 39 sessions, but I was aware that Koreans only receive 28 fractions.

John from Queensland also only had 28 treatments. At that time, we had no real idea how we would enjoy Korea and felt that 39 sessions, together with a number of public holidays, would see us there for 10 weeks, which might drag on somewhat, if we were not enjoying the non-medical side of the visit. Dr Cho indicated that 28 fractions at slightly higher dosage would be more than adequate. They are inclined to do the 39 sessions as that is what the USA and European competitors offer! He also indicated that I would receive a small credit for the accommodation saving, at the end of our stay. So 28 treatments it was to be. I could hardly wait to get started and attack the cancerous cells multiplying in my body. Having said that, the Zoladex® ADT effect had well and truly kicked in, with my testosterone levels and PSA way down. My libido was also close to non-existent, and I told my wife that *"men were starting to look attractive"*! Dr Cho suggested that I have my second Zoladex® injection, when it was due in mid-February.

He indicated that they were well-pleased with my medical records and that my treatment would start on the following Monday. He gave me a full medical including a DRE. He found my prostate to be pressing against my rectal wall but with no irregularities. Pam and I were to meet with Dr Cho each Tuesday until my treatment was concluded. I found him very engaging and felt that his team would deliver me an optimal outcome.

Pam was ushered back to the VIP private room, whilst I was taken by Ms Hyun Ah Lim, their international proton therapy coordinator, to the pathology station to give them a urine sample. As I was a little dehydrated, it was a bit of a challenge. I emerged from the sampling room with the capped bottle of urine in my hand. I was in trouble, as I should have opened a small sliding opaque window and placed the sample on a shelf. Surprisingly, as I finally placed the sample bottle on the shelf, another opaque door opened and a gloved hand removed the sample. By the way, Ms Lim spoke reasonable English.

Following the CT bone scan, I was met by Wendy, who had received our treatment time schedule. The first session was to be at 3.15pm on the Monday, thereafter at 10.30am until the 24th January, when I would move into Henry's time slot of 10am. As I moved into the radiology department for an MRI scan, I met Jan coming out after his MRI. He definitely did not enjoy the claustrophobic experience. Five minutes later it was my turn. Even with headphones on and with piped music, the 45 minute session had continuous loud noises being propagated by the magnet movements. Half way through the MRI, a contrasting agent was injected via the cannula previously inserted in the back of my hand. The hard part was placing my arms above my head for an extended period, whilst breathing in and out on command. The MRI is a very important process in the planning of the treatment program with the prostate image being integrated into the daily x-ray set up procedure. After the MRI, I changed into civvies and Mr Chow drove us back to our apartment, arriving there at 5.45pm after a long, but interesting day.

On returning to our unit, we couldn't get our internet working, nor could Pam get the induction hot top or gas stove top to work. The "engineer" duly arrived at our request, and the internet was soon working. The "engineer" who spoke no English, showed us where to turn the induction hot top on at the mains and the almost secret gas cock on for the stove. Tomorrow, the CT simulation scans are due, starting at 2pm. Pam said *"I'm giving it a miss"*. Mr Chow, who spoke very little English, but had an ability to make himself understood, and with a great sense of humour, delivered me to the NCC safely on time. We were to learn that punctuality was one of his greatest assets.

On the Wednesday morning, Pam and I explored the local area in the cold (-10° C). We bought two Travel Cards at the 24 hour convenience shop in the complex. These allowed us to travel by train, taxi or bus anywhere in Korea. Travel there is very cheap. We discovered that a taxi from the nearest metro station, which was a mile away from our apartment, cost us about $2. Our exploration failed to find either of the two Paris Baguette shops that we were told were "only 5 minutes" walk away. There were numerous coffee shops and restaurants within easy walking distance. We were to find that at least 50 coffee chains exist in Seoul. Many were well known Western brands.

On arrival at the NCC, I was again escorted into the VIP private ward, and given a pair of hospital issue turquoise-coloured thick pyjamas to put on without underpants. I was told a nurse would arrive shortly to do an enema, after which I was to drink 4 glasses of water. This was all accomplished and the cannula re-inserted in my hand. They drew black lines on my upper legs, belly button downwards and crosses adjacent to my hip joints. They then produced a probe that had spikes on the end and inserted it up my rectum. It hurt like hell. It was withdrawn after a few minutes and replaced with another probe/catheter that was left in situ whilst the CT scan was completed. I was then transferred to the hospital radiology department in another building where I had another MRI done with another probe (endorectal coil) up my rectum. Fortunately, the MRI took only 15 minutes, by which time I was bursting to pass urine.

On the way back to the hotel, I spotted the Paris Baguette shop. That's where tomorrow's lunch was coming from. The Thursday and Friday were free days. The medical physicists and doctors used it for:

Computer treatment planning

Pre-treatment quality assurance procedure completion

Manufacture of the block and compensators to be used on the proton beam delivery system.

The two compensators are made out of a hard plastic material. They have a cut-out relief in each which is an exact copy of the shape of one half of the prostate. They are used to minimise the radiation to areas beyond the prostate outer wall. The blocks are solid pieces of brass that are about three inches thick with an aperture in them, with the aperture being the exact outline of the prostate as seen from the hip joint. The right hand block and compensator are replaced by left hand versions as the gantry moves overhead to prepare for the treatment of the other side of the prostate.

By now, Pam and I had mapped out all the places we wanted to visit and the things we wanted to see during our stay. The holiday side of the trip started in earnest. We quickly discovered that Korea was an enchanting place and the people were very helpful and engaging. We estimated that about 20% of the people could speak English, to a greater or lesser extent. You only had to stop on a street corner and look at a map before someone would come up to try to help you. We had a few comical such encounters with people who could speak no English, but were determined to help us. Wearing our thermal underwear, heavy overcoats, gloves, a scarf and headgear, made us more able to cope with the very cold weather.

It became the norm to get back from the NCC at about 11.15am each treatment day, have a hot cup of coffee, put on my thermals and for Pam and I to head off sightseeing. Each day, the apartment complex courtesy bus went to HomePlus and did other set trips down town. Every Saturday, it took us to a Costco and HomePlus near the NCC. We were amazed at the shopping loads that people brought back onto the bus. As the weeks went by, we became very familiar with the local bus service, using green, red or blue buses that passed the DMC Ville every two minutes or so. It cost us about 60 cents each to get to town.

We also developed a good friendship with Henry and Helen. Pam joined them most Sundays at a church in downtown Seoul where they were all made very welcome. Jan's schedule called for afternoon treatment, so we didn't see too much of him, though occasionally we would spend an hour or so comparing notes about our treatment, at one of the coffee shops across the road from the apartments. A few weeks into my treatment, there was general consternation in Seoul, when the regime in North Korea exploded an atomic bomb. A Sunday trip to the Demilitarised Zone between North and South Korea, was a most interesting experience, but made you aware of the continual threat that conflict could resume between these two countries at any time.

Chapter 25.
My Treatment Begins

On the Monday afternoon, I arrived at the PBT Centre in good time and was shown into a change room, where I put on the requisite pyjama trousers without underpants and waited to be called into the treatment room. There are three beam lines at the NCC with one a fixed line that is used for head, eye and neck cancer treatments. I was escorted into the treatment room by the two medical therapists (one spoke good English with the other not so good English). I climbed up on the flat table, removed my pyjama pants, placed my feet up on a type of immobilization device and waited for the balloon catheter to be inserted and filled with water. This took less than a minute to do and the therapists were clearly well skilled in this procedure. The following ten minutes were devoted to positioning me precisely to the millimetre in the correct position. This involves lasers built into the gantry illuminating the crosses previously marked on each hip joint, horizontal and vertical x-ray extensions coming out of the wall to image you in two planes, computer-guided minor adjustment of the table which together matched precisely the position and size of my prostate.

At this point the two therapists left the room to start the diversion of the proton beam through the radiation probe. I could hear the system starting up as it emitted a low whir, which became more intense as the period of radiation started. The proton beam travelling at 100,000 miles per hour irradiated the prostate for about 90 seconds, after which the system went into standby mode. The therapists returned and the gantry moved through 180 degrees to ready itself to irradiate the left side. The right hand block and compensator were replaced with the left hand versions within less than a minute and the same positioning set up was done as for the right-sided entry. The radiation was commenced after the therapists left the room and it was over in no time at all. The rectal catheter was removed and disappeared from view before I could sit up. In fact, I never actually saw it before or after it was inserted all the time I was there. I regained my modesty by pulling my pyjama pants up, climbed off the table, thanked the staff, went to the toilet to do a few running repairs, dressed and was ready to collect Pam and journey back to our apartment. The duration of my time in the treatment room was less than 25 minutes.

This procedure was undertaken time and again. It was totally uneventful, until the good English-speaker was promoted and a new medical therapist joined my treatment team. After a few days as the No. 2 man, it was his turn to insert the balloon catheter. He pushed it in, but didn't know when to stop. A quick screech in pain from me, made him realise that I was running out of room! He was very embarrassed and even more apologetic. I never had a problem after that.

Weekly meetings with Dr Cho, were pleasant experiences, but uneventful. On the second last treatment day, I had blood and urine samples taken. Yes, I used the sliding door and saw the other door open and the urine sample disappear into a gloved hand. On the 21st February, I had my 28th and last fraction. After the session concluded, I was invited to bang the shield (just like the Rank Organisation shield of old movie fame) outside the treatment rooms to signify the end of my journey. This was followed by morning tea with Dr Cho, his medical therapists, the medical physicists, Ms Lim, Wendy and the reliable Mr Chow. Paris Baguette had provided a great cream cake. Dr Cho again thanked me for selecting the NCC for treatment and presented me with a wonderful certificate confirming my attendance at their facility. He also included a USB which included my medical records which confirmed that I had received 7000 cGy, the agreed dose, at the rate of 250 cGy per fraction.

All I had to prove that I had had the treatment was a circular spot about two inches in diameter on each hip joint. This was "sunburn" caused by the entry of the proton beam at this spot. The next morning Mr Chow drove us out to the Incheon International Airport and we thanked him for his service whilst we had been in Seoul. We had two experiences whilst in his care. One morning, we were on our way to the hospital when we hit some black ice. The car spun through 360 degrees without hitting anything and we continued after a laughing apology from Mr Chow. The other 'happening' was the freeway being blocked by South Korean soldiers. We thought hostilities may have started with the crazy North Koreans, who are still technically at war with the South. Apparently, they were on an army manoeuvre. The South Korean people were very perturbed by the Northern Koreans undertaking two atomic bomb tests whilst we were in Seoul. The Demilitarised Zone is only 55 kilometres (34 miles) from Seoul and only 30 kilometres (19 miles) from the NCC. Our one day trip to the DMZ reinforced the threat that the North represent to the South.

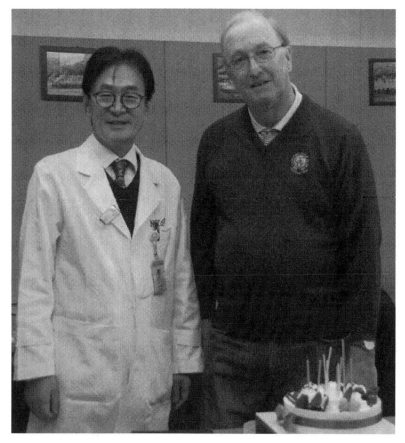

Image: Dr Cho Kwang-Ho and me after my treatment was concluded. Note Paris Baguette cake!

Chapter 26.

The Post-Treatment Period

By the end of April 2013, the last of the Zoladex® had left my system and my hormonal state returned to normal. I certainly stopped looking at the men and noticed pretty girls again! My first PSA after my return to Australia was 0.26 and a subsequent result in June 2014 was 0.22. I have not yet reached the nadir value which should be reached late in 2014. All as one might expect. My free PSA was at 5% versus 9% in early 2012.

In July 2013, the rectal bleeding started. It was only minor, but it was a bit of a shock to have the toilet paper all red for the first time. My general practitioner prescribed a cortisone-based 100ml retention enema to be injected at bedtime each night, but this didn't make any difference to the small, but regular bleeding. It was early January 2014, when I decided to raise the issue with Dr Cho. He responded promptly to the point that only 2 in 10 PBT patients exhibit rectal bleeding and it appeared that I was one of them. As I take warfarin for an arrhythmia problem, the condition is almost self-sustaining. He suggested that I should get my bowel checked by a proctologist or colo-rectal specialist. This I did and it was found that I had a radiation burn the size of the fingernail of a man's smallest finger.

The specialist recommended that we wait four months before deciding on one of the three treatments options used for this condition. I went back to Dr Cho at the NCC with a copy of the photo of the offending area. His response was that it would likely disappear of its own accord over time or I could start a course of rectal retention enemas, with sucralfate as the active ingredient. Unfortunately, it is not possible to get sucralfate in suspension in Australia. However, the good news is that the bleeding had almost stopped and I expected it to be completely gone, within a few weeks. (In fact, after a three month period with no bleeding, it surprisingly returned in July and as of mid-October it still persists). Due to unrelated issues, my physician has changed my daily warfarin dose for a new blood thinner called Rivaroxaban (Xarelto® - Bayer). This change might also help alleviate the bleeding problem. (to date it hasn't - the bleeding continues to be very minor and is completely bearable)

Chapter 27.
Would I make the same Decision Again?

After having researched and written this book, I have learned a great deal more about prostate cancer than I knew when I assessed my treatment options. I was exposed to prostate cancer in the family before my own diagnosis. Even this did not equip me with anywhere near enough information to be able to cope with what outcomes were possible with the various alternative treatments. Whilst I am sure that almost all doctors are well intentioned when they make their recommendations, it's you the patient, who has to live with the consequences of any treatment undertaken. Some people get side effects that nobble them. As reported earlier in the book, I have a friend that did not have a good outcome from a radical prostatectomy. The result was he started to find relief by drinking far too heavily for his own and his family's good.

The simple issue is that men need to take matters into their own hands by intelligently and thoroughly researching the options open to them. Unless they are diagnosed with metastatic cancer which requires immediate action, they have time to weigh up carefully the various options open to them. Remember that prostate cancer, in the main, is a disease that progresses slowly. This leads me to the story that a friend of mine related to me recently.

Rob was about 55 when he was diagnosed with prostate cancer in 2000. Rob continues his story with some comment from me that is in normal type face. *"At the insistence of my general practitioner I had a PSA test 14 years ago. It came back at 460 ng/ml. The GP had already made an appointment with Dr F (a well-known urologist at a prestigious private hospital) and I went along not really knowing the seriousness of the report. I had no symptoms and was very fit. No point in operating as the cancer had already spread and a Gleason Score of 8. Dr F put me on hormone therapy and said if all went well, I might have 3 to 5 years. (Expletive deleted). After about one year my PSA was down to 1 or thereabouts, but started to rise in year two. Tried various other supplementary drugs which slowed growth for a while, but still on the rise. At about year 5, PSA was 23 and increasing quickly. Chemo was recommended. Not for me said I. I think I would like to see Dr Snuffy Myers in the USA (Dr F had advised me to buy his book. I had done so and followed his diet regimen very closely which no doubt had helped a lot. Meanwhile, I had subscribed to his newsletter). My then specialist (Dr F had flick passed me on - a real hospital pass this one) said it was a good idea and he had another patient go to see him with quite positive outcomes. (Why he didn't suggest it himself is a mystery).*

So off to USA and Snuffy. He reckoned for all that my cancer was something of a sheep in wolf's clothing. Came home with a three month course of Leukine (not available here) to be taken in conjunction with Thalidomide®. PSA down to low single figures. Whoopee. After a year or so on the rise again, so Snuffy says start with Ketaconazol® (meant for treatment of fungal infections). Down it goes again, but side effects not pleasant. As time went by had to increase the dose of Ketaconazol® to double that recommended. Felt terrible. After a year or two, PSA at 28. Back to USA. Scans I had didn't show anything, although clearly the cancer was on the march. He had me get scans in Orlando, Florida. And these showed a lesion in my pelvic area - lymph node. Snuffy sent me back with a DVD of the scan and an instruction to contact Dr K at a large Sydney hospital where I had 40 episodes of IMRT. That was 3 1/2 years ago. PSA now 0.02. Still on Zoladex® and Avodart® (which inhibits conversion of Testosterone into Dihydrotesterone - which the cancer feeds on) still watch diet but not as rigorously. Feel great. Radiation damage to bladder has affected my urination a bit but manageable. Up 3 to 5 times a night, but who cares".

I include this story as a true inspiration to those with a challenging prognosis for their prostate cancer. I also include it as it shows that no matter how dire is the prognosis, much can be done by the patient himself taking the initiative and finding the best medical help available. It may not be on your doorstep. It might be somewhere else in the world. Sure monetary considerations come into it, but in some cases, it's your life you are playing with. Rob is fit and reasonably well more than 9 years after he was supposed to be dead, because he investigated options not initially put forward by his doctors.

What would I do differently, with what I know now, compared with what information I had available to me, when I made the decision to go to have proton beam therapy in Korea?

In essence, nothing different.

I would still have opted to go to Korea for treatment. However, there are a lot of "ifs" that arise.

If I had not had the TURP procedure that excluded me from having transurethral hyperthermia treatment together with a series of biological cocktails to help kill the cancer, I would have opted for that alternative. It was a rapid and inexpensive treatment, which would not exclude me from having almost all other treatments as a salvage procedure.

If I had known more about mpMRI and colour Doppler ultrasound earlier, I would have insisted on having both done. It would have shown up the precise size, position and extent of the tumours in my prostate. This knowledge may have allowed me to consider treatment of these tumours alone by focussed technologies like HIFU or FLA. This may have left part of my prostate active.

If my Gleason Score was 6 (versus the actual 7), I would have gone onto an active surveillance regime, with mpMRI and Power Doppler ultrasound providing progress reports on the tumour growth.

If I had much more knowledge of the effectiveness of the latest radiation devices such as RapidArc® and IMRT, I just might have gone down the treatment course of high dose brachytherapy followed by radiation provided by either of these systems.

If I could have found a top surgeon using the da Vinci® prostatectomy system with an exemplary record of nerve sparing outcomes, I might have gone down that path, as a radical prostatectomy offers better choices should there be a recurrence of the cancer.

If I had not been "scared to death" of having malignant cells growing in my body which I needed killing immediately, I would have gone into far greater depth in my research efforts.

If I had been fully familiar with the SpaceOAR® hydrogel before my radiation treatment, I would have had the rectum sparing injection. In Australia the cost is covered by medical insurance.

However, life is all about the here and now and "ifs" need to be put into their place as a past opportunity, perhaps a good one, lost. Or more likely, perhaps a lesser outcome being achieved.

So I can confirm that I would again select proton beam therapy treatment at the National Cancer Centre in Korea as the best alternative to suit my unique circumstances. Of course, to select Proton Beam Therapy, without any health insurance reimbursement, puts PBT beyond the financial reach of most families. Perhaps the same can be said of a few of the other treatments considered in this book. The capability of families to access (geographically, financially or medically) any form of treatment is as variable as the human condition. Readers of this book, each with their own circumstances, might feel similarly or opt for a different course of treatment.

I predict that mpMRI together with focal laser treatment will transform the prostate cancer treatment field for low and intermediate risk patients over the next few years. I also predict that the Holy Grail of finding a treatment that offers few side effects and the lowest recurrence rates will be achieved before 2025.

A final word. I have written this book to try to fill in the many blanks that existed in my knowledge of prostate cancer when I had to decide on a course of action. I will be well pleased if I have been able to help even one prostate cancer sufferer. Hopefully, it will be of assistance to many. Much of the material that I have researched for this book has come from discussions with my doctors, fellow sufferers, a host of books read on the subject and by spending hundreds of hours on the internet. I doubt that there is more information available on any other disease than that available for prostate cancer.

I have said many times in this book that **I am NOT a doctor**, and have stressed that it is imperative that you consult your medical team at each and every opportunity so that you can jointly develop a treatment program that optimises outcomes for you. Hopefully, the questions that I have listed in this book, (and others not listed by me) for you to ask your doctors, might lead to you being as well informed as possible as you undertake your fight back to good health.

I feel that my "journey" over four continents to find the "best" cure has been a success as far as my treatment is concerned. I thank you for reading this book, and if you are so inclined, refer it to others who might be inflicted with prostate cancer, so that they might have more knowledge available to them. After all knowledge is power. I wish you well.

THE END.

Appendix 1

Glossary

acidosis
An abnormal condition resulting from the accumulation of acid or the depletion of alkalis in the body.

active surveillance
A management option for localized prostate cancer patients with the intent to intervene if the disease progresses as revealed by regular testing.

adjuvant therapy
A treatment given in conjunction with or shortly after another treatment to enhance its effectiveness.

advanced prostate cancer
Prostate cancer that has spread to neighbouring tissues or to other parts of the body.

alternative therapy
Monotherapies whose efficacy has not been validated by clinical trials.

anaesthetic
A drug given to stop a person feeling pain. A local anaesthetic numbs part of the body; a general anaesthetic causes temporary lack of consciousness.

androgens
Male sex hormones. The most active male hormone, testosterone, is produced by the testicles. Other male hormones are produced by the adrenal glands.

androgen deprivation therapy (ADT)
A drug treatment that minimises the effect of testosterone in the body. This type of therapy can slow or stop the growth of prostate cancer. Also called androgen suppression therapy.

androgen suppression therapy (AST)
See ADT.

androgen synthesis inhibitors (ASI)
Compounds with characteristics that are likely to provide effective antitumor activity against androgen dependent prostatic cancer.

angiogenesis
The ability that tumours have to develop their own blood supply, which helps them to survive and grow.

antigen
Short for antibody generator. They are molecules that provoke an immune response in the body.

anti-androgens
Drugs which slow the growth of prostate cancer by blocking the action of the male hormone, testosterone, in the prostate.

anus
The opening at the end of the rectum through which faeces leaves the body.

apex
The bottom of the prostate.

apical region
The area adjacent to the bottom of the prostate.

ATP
Adenosine triphosphate is a chemical compound that breaks down to release the energy responsible for muscle contraction.

beta-sitosterol
β-sitosterol is used in herbal therapy, especially for benign prostatic hyperplasia (BPH) in a number of countries. It can have potentially serious side effects.

benign
Not cancerous or malignant.

benign prostate enlargement
Non-cancerous enlargement of the prostate which is caused by a condition known as benign hyperplasia (BPH).

benign prostatic hyperplasia
A benign increase in the size of the prostate.

biochemical recurrence
It is the increase in prostate-specific antigen (PSA) in patients after surgery or radiation. It may occur in patients without symptoms. It suggests that the cancer has re-emerged.

bisphosphonate treatment
It assists in the prevention and treatment of osteoporosis, and bone metastasis in patients with metastatic prostate cancer.

biopsy
When prostate cancer is suspected, after a DRE and/or PSA test, tissue samples in the form of rods, are taken from different areas of the prostate, and are then examined under the microscope to see if they are cancerous.

bladder
The organ that stores urine from the kidneys.

bone scan
A nuclear scanning test in which a radioactive chemical is injected, then its path is traced through the body. The chemical concentrates in areas where there is increased bone activity such as areas of cancer, infection or arthritis. Bone scans are not always precise, but are good indicators of cancer cells being present.

boost therapy
The simultaneous or sequential use of a second therapy to boost the overall treatment result.

bovine tracheal cartilage
It is a nutritional supplement that has been claimed to have beneficial outcomes for some prostate cancer sufferers. The cartilage is said to block the formation of new blood vessels which starve tumours of food.

brachytherapy
It is radiotherapy given from within the prostate. Low dose rate brachytherapy involves the permanent insertion of radioactive seeds directly into the prostate. High dose rate brachytherapy involves the temporary insertion of radioactive-tipped needles into the prostate.

Bragg peak effect
The proton radiation increases its energy as it nears its target depth where it releases its maximum energy before it rapidly returns to zero energy.

cancer
Involves abnormal cell growth with the potential to spread to other parts of the body.

cancer anxiety factor
The psychological stress and disposition that develops when a patient is informed that he has cancer.

catechin
Unfermented green teas contain 27% of catechin which interacts with various human genes.

catheter
A hollow, flexible tube through which fluids can be passed into the body or drained from it.

cells
They are the smallest units of life that can independently self-replicate. Cancer cells are abnormal or damaged cells.

chemotherapy
The killing of cancer cells with cytotoxic chemicals. (Cytotoxic means toxic to cells).

clear margin
Also called surgical margin. Usually refers to the visible normal tissue margin that is removed with the surgical removal of a tumour.

clinical staging
It is based on all the available information obtained before surgery to remove a tumour. It may include information about the tumour obtained by physical or radiologic examination. Pathological staging refers to the information obtained by the microscope evaluation by the pathologist.

clinical trial
A trial of a new treatment or drug, conducted by medical researchers on patients who volunteer to take part. These trials are required to be done ethically and in conformity with accepted international principles.

combined modality therapy
The use of more than one therapy at once, often used for high-risk cancers. Therapies may include surgery, radiotherapy, hormone therapy and chemotherapy.

complementary therapy
It is alternative medicine used together with conventional medical treatment with a view that it 'complements' the conventional treatment. The alternative medicine is not proven by scientific research.

computerised tomography (CT) scan
An x-ray scan of a part of the body or region that produce tomographic images or "virtual slices" of the scanned area.

conformal radiotherapy (3D-CRT)
An improved type of external beam radiotherapy (EBRT) where the radiotherapy dose is delivered by a number of beams shaped so that the region where they overlap is similar to the shape of the prostate. This minimises the dose to adjacent healthy tissue.

CyberKnife® radiotherapy
Another variant of conformal radiotherapy. The two main elements are the radiation produced from a small linear accelerator and the use of a robotic arm which allows the energy to be directed at any part of the body from any direction. It reduces the radiation dose to normal tissues, with all parts of the cancer receiving the same dose of radiation.

cryotherapy
A method of killing cancerous cells by freezing the tissue.

cystoscopy
A procedure in which an instrument is introduced along the urethra under local or general anaesthetic, to view the bladder and prostate.

cytotoxicity
The quality of being toxic to cells.

da Vinci® prostatectomy system
A robotic system for complex surgery using a minimally invasive approach.

digital rectal examination (DRE)
An examination of the prostate through the rectum wall. The doctor inserts a finger into the rectum and feels the shape of the prostate, for lumps or areas of hardness which may suggest cancer is present.

dihydrotestosterone (DHT)
DHT, as it is known, has 2 to 3 times the affinity to androgen receptors than testosterone. It has 15 to 30 times more affinity than adrenal androgens. About 5% of testosterone is converted into DHT by the body. DHT is a key food source for cancer cells.

Doppler ultrasound
A medical device that makes use of the Doppler effect to measure and visualise the flow of blood in the prostate.

doubling time
The time taken for the PSA level to double, for example, from 4ng/mL to 8ng/ml. It is a measure of how fast the cancer is growing.

dry ejaculation
After a radical prostatectomy, a man may achieve orgasm, but produce no ejaculate (fluid). This is because the glands that produce most of the fluid are removed. See also reverse ejaculation. The same condition usually exists after a full course of radiation as the "muscles" of the prostate are killed by the radiation.

EBRT
External beam radiation therapy.

ejaculate
Fluid produced at ejaculation, which contains sperm and secretions from the prostate, seminal vesicles and testicles.

EPIC
A questionnaire called the Expanded Prostate Cancer Index Composite (EPIC) requests the patient to quantify against provided criteria, levels of urinary function, bowel activities, sexual function and overall satisfaction post treatment.

erectile dysfunction
The inability to achieve an erection firm enough for penetration.

erection
When the penis becomes enlarged and rigid during and after arousal.

oestrogens
They are the primary female sex hormones.

external beam radiation (EBRT)
X-ray-based radiotherapy given from a source external of the body.

extra capsular extension
Cancer that extends through the capsule of the prostate into the surrounding tissue, as determined from the radical prostatectomy pathology report.

FACT-P
Functional Assessment of Cancer Therapy-Prostate (FACT-P) is a multidimensional, self-reported Quality of Life questionnaire specifically designed for use with prostate cancer patients.

faecal incontinence
Involuntary loss of faeces.

fertility
The ability to naturally conceive children.

fiducial marker
A non-radioactive marker (often gold seeds) inserted in the prostate to accurately locate it. It is part of the radiotherapy planning process and helps the accuracy of image-guided radiotherapy (IGRT).

five-year survival rate
A scientific measure to determine the success of a treatment, because it is hard to know if someone is cured or simply in remission. It measures the number of people who are alive after a particular treatment.

focal laser ablation (FLA)
The removal or ablation of diseased tissue by the focused heat energy of a laser.

free to total PSA ratio
The prostate-specific antigen (PSA) in the bloodstream can "latch" onto protein. This is called "bound" PSA. In men with BPH, there tends to be more "free" or "unbound" PSA. This test compares the ratio of unbound PSA to total PSA in the bloodstream.

gene
The tiny factors that govern the way the body's cells grow and behave. Each person has many thousand of genes inherited from both parents and they are found in every cell.

ginseng (Panax variety)
Panax ginsengs are herbs that have pharmacological properties. Their alternative therapy efficacies have not been proven in clinical studies.

Gleason score
A method of grading cancer cells. Low grade cancers with Gleason scores of 2, 3, or 4 grow slower than high grade (Gleason scores 8, 9, or 10) cancers. The pathologist identifies the two most common tissue patterns under a microscope and grades them from 1 (least aggressive) to 5 (most aggressive). The Gleason score is given as two numbers added together to give a score out of 10 (for example, 3 + 4 = 7). The first number is the most common pattern present and the second number is the next most common.

glutamine
It is the most abundant non-essential amino acid in the body. It has therapeutic properties when taken as a food supplement.

grade/grading
A score which describes the level of abnormality of cancer cells, and consequently how aggressive or fast-growing the cancer is likely to be. The most commonly used grading system is the Gleason score, which ranges from 2 to 10 (see above).

gray (Gy)
A measure of a dose of ionizing radiation. A gray is defined as the absorption of one joule of radiation energy by one kilogram of matter.

HDR remote after-loader
A medical device used in HDR brachytherapy which automatically 'loads' the radioactive tipped needles and stores them safely.

high dose rate brachytherapy
HDR brachytherapy is a temporary radiation treatment for cancer and the amount of time that the radiation source is left in place is determined by the radiation oncologist.

high intensity focused ultrasound (HIFU)
It is a highly precise medical procedure that applies high-intensity focused ultrasound energy to locally heat and destroy diseased or damaged tissue through ablation.

homeopathy
A system of alternative medicine in which a substance that causes the symptoms of a disease in healthy people will cure similar symptoms in sick people.

hormones
Natural bio-chemical substances that are produced by one body organ, and travel through the bloodstream to other organs where they influence its physiology and behaviour.

hormone resistance
Prostate cancer cells are dependent on testosterone growth. Withdrawal of testosterone by surgery or by means of drugs is therefore a means of controlling its growth. However, cancer cells may develop which do not need testosterone for growth. The cancer is then said to be "hormone resistant".

hot flushes
A sudden feeling of heat to the face, neck, chest and back that usually lasts for a few minutes, but can continue for an hour. It is brought about by prostate cancer hormone therapy.

hyperbaric oxygen
Oxygen delivered at above atmospheric pressure. It can be helpful in relieving some long-term side effects of radiation such as rectal bleeding.

hyperthermia
It is a type of cancer treatment in which body tissue is exposed to high temperatures (up to 43°C or 113°F). There are various formats, such as, regional, transurethral and whole body hyperthermia.

hypoxia, hypoxemia
Hypoxia: a condition in which the body or a region of the body is deprived of adequate oxygen supply.
Hypoxemia: insufficient oxygenation of arterial blood.

IIEF-15
The International Index of Erectile Function-15 is a standard set of 15 questions that was developed as a measure to detect treatment-related erectile function in patients.

image-guided radiotherapy (IGRT)
Radiotherapy guided by specialised imaging tests, such as CT scans, ultrasound or x-rays. These tests are done in the treatment room just before the patient is to receive daily radiation treatment or during the radiation delivery to compensate for movement of the prostate.

impotence
See erectile dysfunction.

immune-therapeutical agents
They are inhibitors of tumour necrosis factor α.

incidental finding
The discovery of cancerous tissue during other procedures, like a TURP.

incontinence
The involuntary passing of urine (urinary incontinence) or faeces (faecal incontinence).

indolent
A type of cancer cells that grow very slowly.

infertility
The inability to conceive naturally.

intensity modulated radiotherapy (IMRT)
A type of conformal external beam radiotherapy where the radiotherapy dose is delivered by dozens of mini-beams of radiation. IMRT usually results in less radiation dose to normal tissues, whilst all parts of the cancer receiving the same dose of radiation.

intermittent hormone therapy
Hormone therapy which is started and stopped in cycles. Typically, it is continued for several months until the PSA has declined to a low level, and then discontinued. Once the PSA level rises to a particular level again, which might take many months, hormone therapy is restarted. This approach reduces side effects during the 'off ' period.

interstitial
Situated within an organ or tissue.

IPSS
The International Prostate Symptom Score (IPSS) is an 8 question written screening tool to screen, diagnose and manage the treatment of BPH.

irreversible electroporation #
It is a soft tissue ablation technique using ultra short but strong electrical fields to create permanent nanopores in the cell membrane. The resulting cell death results from apoptosis.

Kattan nomogram
A tool that predicts prostate cancer progression outcomes - whether they are for those initially diagnosed or all degrees of the disease to the metastatic stage.

lactoferrin
It is a multifunctional protein of the transferrin family and it is a component of the immune system of the body which has antimicrobial activity and is part of the innate defence of the body.

laparoscopic surgery
A surgical method where the operation is performed using small incisions through thin telescopic instruments: A small video camera is inserted. The technique is often referred to as 'key-hole' surgery.

LHRH (luteinizing hormone releasing hormone)
A hormone produced by the hypothalamus in the brain and stimulates the pituitary (another part of the brain) to produce LH (luteinizing hormone). This, in turn, causes the testicles to produce the male hormone, testosterone.

LHRH agonists
Drugs that interfere with the production of LH.

LHRH antagonists
Synthetic peptides that interact with gonadotropin-releasing hormone receptor to elicit the release of pituitary hormones FSH and LH.

libido
Sex drive.

localised prostate cancer
Early stage prostate cancer which has not spread beyond the prostate.

locally advanced prostate cancer
Cancer which has spread beyond the prostate capsule and may include the seminal vesicles, but is confined to the prostate or nearby tissues only. Type T3c.

locally recurrent
Cancer that has recurred (come back) after treatment, but which is confined to the prostate or nearby tissue only.

lower urinary tract symptoms (LUTS)
Symptoms related to the flow or passing of urine, such as poor stream, frequent urination, needing to get up at night two or more times to urinate, incontinence and incomplete emptying of the bladder. They are often caused by BPH of the prostate, but can also be caused by advanced prostate cancer.

low dose rate brachytherapy
An internal radiation procedure in which radioactive seeds are permanently implanted in the prostate. They lose their radioactive 'charge' after 6 to 9 months depending on the half-life of the radio-isotope used.

lycopene
It is a carotene found in tomatoes and other 'red' vegetables and has been considered a potential agent for prevention of prostate cancer. The US FDA suggests its efficacy is unproven.

lymph nodes
Also known as lymph glands. They are small, generally pea-sized pieces of tissue found all over the body including the groin area adjacent to the prostate. They act as filters for foreign substances and can harbour cancer cells that have spread from the prostate or elsewhere.

magnetic resonance imaging (MRI)
A machine that produces images of the inside of the body using magnetic forces, without using x-rays.

malignant
Cancerous.

margin positive
When cancer cells are still present at the cutting edge (margin) of the removed prostate after surgery. A negative margin suggests that cancer cells are not present at the cutting edge as determined by a pathologist.

medical oncologist
A specialist in the treatment of cancer using chemotherapy.

metastasis/metastasise
The spread of cancer away from the place where it began.

metastatic prostate cancer
Cancer that has spread from the prostate to the pelvic bones and/or to other organs of the body.

micro-vesicles (cMV's)
They are also called exosomes, circulating micro-vesicles, or micro-particles and are microscopic fragments of plasma membrane shed from almost all cell types. They have been implicated in the process of an anti-tumour reversal effect in cancer, tumour immune suppression, metastasis, and angiogenesis along with having a primary role in tissue regeneration.

Mi-Prostate Score (MIPS)
The MiPS test is an early detection test (pre-biopsy) for prostate cancer that combines the amount of serum PSA, with the amounts of two genes in the urine.

molecular imaging biomarkers
Probes known as biomarkers are used in molecular imaging to help image particular targets or pathways.

monitoring
The process in which patients are subjected to follow up tests and/or clinical examination after the conclusion of initial diagnosis and treatment.

monotherapy
The treatment of cancer by using one form of therapy.

multiparametric MRI (mpMRI)
It is used to better identify and characterize prostate cancer. When T2-weighted, dynamic contrast enhanced, and diffusion-weighted imaging were used together the specificity and sensitivity for finding clinically significant prostate cancer (a Gleason score of 6 or higher and size exceeding 5 millimeters) was between 85 percent and 96 percent.

nadir
The lowest PSA reading reached after treatment for prostate cancer, before the PSA starts to rise again. This can occur some months after radiotherapy to cure prostate cancer.

neo-adjuvant therapy
Treatment given before another treatment to enhance its effectiveness.

neo-vascularity
The formation of a microvascular blood supply to feed a tumour.

nerve-sparing operation
Surgery for prostate cancer which aims to preserve the nerves which are essential for erections. The technique is not always possible as cancer can affect the areas around the nerves.

nomogram
Factors such as PSA, grade and stage are combined in a mathematical expression in order to predict outcomes such as the return of the cancer.

oncologist
A specialist in the treatment of cancer (see medical oncologist and radiation oncologist).

orchiectomy (sometimes called orchidectomy)
An operation that removes the testicles, but leaves the scrotal sac or scrotum.

osteoporosis
Literally means "porous bones." It occurs when bones lose a significant amount of their protein and mineral content, particularly calcium.

palliative care
Care of persons whose disease is not responsive to curative treatment. The goal of palliative care is achievement of the best possible quality of life for the person and their family.

pelvis
The area of the body located below the waist and surrounded by the hip and pubic bones.

pelvic floor muscles
These support the bladder and rectum and assist with stress incontinence by giving support to the bladder when coughing or sneezing.

pencil beam scanning
It is the movement of a charged particle beam such as a proton beam, where one or more properties of the beam such as intensity, size or position, are changed to ensure the delivery of the prescribed radiation dose.

penile plethysmograph
A medical device that measures the flow of blood in the penis.

penis
The male reproductive organ.

perineal (perineum)
The area of the body between the anus and the scrotum.

photodynamic therapy #
It is a form of phototherapy using nontoxic light-sensitive compounds that are exposed selectively to light, whereupon they become toxic to targeted malignant and other diseased cells.

pituitary
The part of the brain that produces hormones which stimulate the testicles to produce testosterone.

potency
The ability to have and maintain erections firm enough for penetration.

primary cancer
The original cancer. Cells from the primary cancer may migrate to other parts of the body, where secondary cancers might form.

prognosis
The likely development and outcome of a disease, as estimated by one's doctors.

prostatectomy
A surgical operation to remove all or part of the prostate.

prostate cancer
Localised: cancer confined within the prostate;
Locally advanced: contained within the prostate region and may include the seminal vesicles;
Advanced: cancer that has spread to adjacent organs such as the bladder, rectum and pelvic wall;
Metastatic: cancer that has spread to distant parts of the body.

prostate cancer risk calculator
A system that manually or on line, tallies responses to questions that determine the expected diagnosis type and stage of prostate cancer.

prostate gland
The gland that sits just below the bladder and opens into the urethra. It produces a fluid that forms part of semen. It is referred to in this book as the prostate.

prostate-specific antigen (PSA)
A protein produced by prostate cells, which is usually found in the blood in larger than normal amounts when prostate cancer is present. It is used as a test for prostate cancer or to monitor its recurrence.

prostatitis
Inflammation of the prostate brought about by an infection (or sometimes other causes).

proton beam therapy (PBT)
A type of conformal external beam radiotherapy which uses a beam of protons (instead of x-rays) to irradiate cancerous tissue. PBT reduces the radiation dose to normal tissue, with all parts of the cancer receiving the same radiation dose.

PSA bounce
A temporary rise in PSA reading experienced during the months after brachytherapy to cure prostate cancer. The cause is not well understood.

PSA density
A calculation that compares the PSA value with the size of the prostate which is measured by MRI or ultrasound.

PSA doubling time (PSADT)
The time it takes for the PSA result to double in value.

PSA velocity
How quickly the PSA level rises over time. It is a very important indicator as to the growth of the tumour.

quality of life
The appraisal of your situation and your well-being.

radiation
Energy in the form of waves or particles, including x-rays. This energy can injure or destroy cells by damaging their genetic material, which sees apostates (cell death) occur.

radiation oncologist
A specialist in the treatment of cancer using radiation techniques.

radical prostatectomy
An operation which removes the prostate, part of the urethra, a small part of both vas deferens and the seminal vesicles. This is usually done through a cut in the abdomen.

radical perineal prostatectomy (RPP)
A surgical procedure wherein the prostate gland is removed through an incision in the area between the anus and the scrotum (perineum).

radical retropubic prostatectomy (RRP)
A surgical procedure in which the prostate gland is removed through an incision in the abdomen.

radiotherapy
The use of radiation like x-rays or protons, to kill cancer cells.

RapidArc®
A new advanced non-surgical radiation therapy that destroys tumours using image-guided technology.

rectum
The last part of the bowel, leading to the anus, through which faeces pass. The posterior of the prostate is immediately adjacent to the rectal wall.

recurrence
The re-occurrence of cancer some years after it was first treated.

remission
A term used to describe that there is no sign of cancer after treatment has concluded. It is not necessarily the same as 'cure', as any cancer cells present might not be discovered. In partial remission, some evidence of cancer still remains.

response
A change in the size or extent of the disease due to treatment.

reverse (or retrograde) ejaculation
This may occur after surgery for benign conditions of the prostate. The ejaculate travels back into the bladder instead of exiting through the penis. This means a man is usually infertile, but an orgasm is still possible.

robot-assisted laparoscopic prostatectomy (RALP)
Minimally invasive surgery to remove the prostate. Small cuts are made in the abdomen. Surgery is conducted using telescopic instruments inserted through these cuts and controlled remotely by the surgeon with the aid of computerised 'robot'.

salvage treatment
Further treatment to try to destroy cancer cells that survived the initial treatment and have since multiplied significantly. A form of radiation is usually used.

saw palmetto
As an extract, it is used by men with BPH. Clinical trials have not confirmed its efficacy, but it has a large following.

stereotactic beam radiation therapy (SBRT)
SBRT involves the delivery of a single high dose radiation treatment or a few fractionated radiation treatments (usually up to 5 treatments). The radiation is delivered using a specially designed coordinate-system that precisely monitors the location of fiducial markers implanted in the tumour before the radiation begins. This specialized form of radiation involves the use of multiple radiation beam angles to maximise the radiation dose to the tumour whilst minimising radiation to adjacent healthy tissue.

screening
Testing an at-risk population for a medical condition, to find people who have the condition, although obvious symptoms are not yet evident.

scrotum
A pouch of skin which hangs behind the penis and contains the testicles and some other parts of the male reproductive system.

secondary cancer
See metastasis.

semen
The fluid ejaculated from the penis at sexual climax.

seminal vesicles
Glands adjacent to the prostate that produce secretions which form part of the ejaculate.

shark cartilage
It is a dietary supplement made from the dried and powdered cartilage of a shark. It has been claimed that it provides therapeutic benefits when used for treating prostate cancer.

stage/staging
A system for describing how far the cancer has spread. The most common is the TNM system with T standing for the tumour size; Nfor lymph nodes and M for metastasis.

stress incontinence
Uncontrolled loss of a small amount of urine as a result of laughing, coughing, sneezing or any strenuous activity, such as lifting heavy objects.

stricture
When urine flow is obstructed by a narrowing of the urethra by injury or disease.

surgery
An operation or a medical procedure involving an incision or cut in order to investigate or treat a medical condition.

surgical margin
After a radical prostatectomy, the edges of the tissue that has been removed are visually examined to see if cancer cells are present. If they are not (negative surgical margins) the chance is higher that all of the cancer has been removed. A pathologist often reviews the removed tissue to check the surgical margin for remaining cancer.

survival
Prostate cancer specific: the proportion of men who survive for a given period, say five years.
Biochemical: the proportion of men surviving without an increase in PSA levels for a given period, say five years.

testicles
Organs in the scrotum which produce sperm and the male hormone, testosterone.

testosterone
The major male hormone which is mainly produced by the testicles.

testosterone flare
The surge in testosterone levels that is seen when treating patients with GnRH agonists.

tissue
A collection of cells.

TNM system
The TNM Classification of Malignant Tumours is a cancer staging system that describes the extent of a person's cancer.
T describes the size of the original (primary) tumour and whether it has invaded nearby tissue.
N describes nearby (regional) lymph nodes that are involved.
M describes distant metastasis (spread of cancer from one part of the body to another).

tomo therapy
A type of radiation therapy in which the radiation is delivered slice-by-slice. This method of delivery differs from other forms of external beam radiation therapy in which the entire tumour volume is irradiated at one time.

transrectal ultrasound (TRUS)
Used for the evaluation of the prostate in men with elevated PSA or prostatic nodules on DRE. It may reveal prostate cancer, BPH, or prostatitis and its imaging capability is also used to help guide a prostate biopsy needle. The ultrasound probe is inserted in the rectum.

transurethral resection of the prostate (TURP)
An operation for BPH of the prostate, but sometimes used to treat prostate cancer. An instrument is inserted, under anaesthetic, along the urethra and removes prostate tissue which may be blocking the flow of urine.

tumour
Any abnormal growth of tissue which may be benign or cancerous

urethra
The tube which carries urine and ejaculate along the length of the penis and then to exit the body.

uroflowmetry
Free uroflowmetry test: measures how fast the patient can empty his bladder.
Pressure uroflowmetry test: measures the rate of voiding, and simultaneous assessment of bladder and rectal pressures.

urologist
A medical specialist who diagnoses and treats urological conditions.

vas deferens
Ducts that take sperm to the urethra on ejaculation.

watchful waiting
An approach to low grade prostate cancer where medical intervention or therapy is delayed until repeat testing may suggest the need for intervention.

whole body hyperthermia
A medical treatment in which the body is exposed to elevated temperatures that kill cancer cells, whilst doing no damage to healthy cells.

x-ray
A form of electromagnetic radiation.

\# This terminology is included for completeness. Details are not included in the general text of the book.

Appendix 2.
Abbreviations

3D-CRT	conformal radiotherapy
ADT	androgen deprivation therapy
ASI	androgen synthesis inhibitors
ASTRO	American Soc. for Therapeutic Radiology and Oncology
ATP	adenosine triphosphate
AUA	American Urological Association
BPH	benign prostate hypertrophy
CIPC	clinically insignificant prostate cancer
CNS	central nervous system
CRCP	metastatic castration-resistant prostate cancer
CT	computerised tomography
DCE-MRI	dynamic contrast enhanced MRI
DHT	dihydrotestosterone
DNA	deoxyribonucleic acid
DRE	digital rectal examination
DW-MRI	diffusion-weighted MRI
EBRT	external beam radiation therapy
EPIC	Expanded Prostate Cancer Index Composite
FACT-P	Functional Assessment of Cancer Therapy - Prostate
FDA	US Food and Drug Administration
FLA	focal laser ablation
Gy	gray
HCL	Harvard Cyclotron Laboratory
HDR	HDR brachytherapy
HIFU	high intensity focused ultrasound
IGRT	image-guided radiotherapy
IIEF-15	The International Index of Erectile Function-15
IMPT	intensity modulated proton therapy
IMRT	intensity modulated radiotherapy
IPSS	The International Prostate Symptom Score
KMI	Korean Medical International
LDR	LDR brachytherapy

Abbreviations (Continued)

LLUMC	Loma Linda University Medical Centre
MHz	megahertz
MiPS	Mi-Prostate Score
mpMRI	multiparametric MRI
MRI	magnetic resonance imaging
NCC	National Cancer Centre, South Korea
NCCN	US National Comprehensive Cancer Network
NHA	new generation hormonal agents
PBT	proton beam therapy
PET	positron emission tomography
PI-RADS	Prostate Imaging Reporting and Data System
PSADT	PSA doubling time
RALP	robot-assisted laparoscopic prostatectomy
RCT	randomised clinical trials
RF	radio frequency
RNA	ribonucleic acid
RPP	radical perineal prostatectomy
RRP	radical retropubic prostatectomy
SBRT	stereotactic beam radiation therapy
TCM	traditional Chinese medicine
TGA	Australian Therapeutic Goods Administration
TRUS	transrectal ultrasound
TUH	transurethral hyperthermia
TURP	transurethral resection of the prostate
UCL	University College of London
UCLA	University of California of Los Angeles
UCLH	University College of London Hospital
USPSTF	US Preventitive Services Task Force
WBH	whole body hyperthermia

Appendix 3.

Resource Listing

Chapter 2. What is Prostate Cancer?
Booklet: "Living with bone metastases from prostate cancer".
http://www.prostate.org.au/articleLive/pages/All-Publications.html#Brochures.

Chapter 3. How is Prostate Cancer detected?
The USPSTF full report.
http://www.uspreventiveservicestaskforce.org/prostatecancerscreening/prostatefinalrs.htm

The USPSTF one page summary report.
http://www.uspreventiveservicestaskforce.org/prostatecancerscreening/prostatecancerinfo.pdf.

The AUA new PSA testing guidelines.
https://www.auanet.org/education/guidelines/prostate-cancer-detection.cfm

Interesting Questions and Answers on MiPS.
http://www.mlabs.umich.edu/files/pdfs/MiPS_FAQ.pdf

More information on mpMRI and prostate cancer.
http://www.cancernetwork.com/prostate-cancer/state-prostate-mri-2013/page/0/1#sthash.5i1qxGq6.dpuf.

UCLA combines the use of an MRI with advanced Doppler ultrasound technology to produce a 3D "fusion" image. See video.
http://urology.ucla.edu/body.cfm?id=455.

Details of the Tissue Harmonic technology with Colour Doppler TRUS practiced by Dr. Duke Bahn, Prostate Institute of America.
http://pioa.org/about-prostate-cancer/accurate-staging/color-doppler-tissue-harmonic-ultrasound/

PCPTR2.0 Calculator
http://deb.uthscsa.edu/URORiskCalc/Pages/calcs.jsp

Sunnybrook Prostate Cancer Risk Calculator
http://sunnybrook.ca/content/?page=occ-prostateriskca.

Chapter 5. Watchful Waiting or Active Surveillance
The US National Comprehensive Cancer Network has recently updated their Prostate Cancer Guidelines.
http://www.nccn.org/patients/guidelines/prostate/index.html#1.

PSA doubling time (PSADT) is a very important parameter in judging the degree of aggressiveness of the cancer. http://prostate-cancer.org/active-surveillance-for-favorable-risk-prostate-cancer-what-are-the-results-and-how-safe-is-it/

Chapter 6. Surgery
da Vinci® Surgery Web Site http://www.davincisurgery.com/da-vinci-urology/conditions/prostate-cancer/da-vinci-prostatectomy/

The da Vinci® Surgery web site compares patient outcomes for open, laparoscopic and da Vinci® RALP surgery.
http://www.davincisurgery.com/da-vinci-urology/treatment-comparison/da-vinci-vs-open-lap.php

Chapter 7.1 External Beam Radiation Therapy SpaceOAR® System – Spacing Organs At Risk.
http://www.augmenix.com/products/spaceoar/.

Chapter 7.4 Proton Beam Therapy
A paper: "Proton beam therapy and localized prostate cancer: current status and controversies".
http://www.nature.com/bjc/journal/v108/n6/full/bjc2013100a.html.

Chapter 7.5 Low Dose Rate Brachytherapy (Seeds)
An excellent web site on LDR brachytherapy.
http://www.cancerresearchuk.org/cancer-help/type/prostate-cancer/treatment/radiotherapy/internal-radiotherapy-for-prostate-cancer#quick

Chapter 8. Hyperthermia
Further details on non-local hyperthermia.
http://en.wikipedia.org/wiki/Hyperthermia_therapy#Mechanism.

Chapter 9. Cryosurgery
Best Practice Policy Statement on Cryosurgery for the Treatment of Localized Prostate Cancer.
http://www.auanet.org/education/guidelines/cryosurgery.cfm.

Chapter 13. Chemotherapy and Immunotherapy
An excellent pictorial illustration of the path to successful immunotherapy discovery and treatment.
www.cancerresearch.org/cancer-immunotherapy/what-is-cancer-immunotherapy.

When prostate cancer continues to grow treatment options become more limited. http://www.cancerresearch.org/prostate-cancer#sthash.IP5NLb41.dpuf.

Caris Life Sciences profiling service. www.carislifesciences.com

Chapter 14. Complementary and Alternative Therapies
Dr Charles "Snuffy" Myers Prostate Forum.
http://www.prostateforum.com/overview.html

"Promaxin Ultimate" is available from Medicines from Nature.
http://www.medicinesfromnature.com.au/pmu.html

Ron Gellatley's books.
http://www.health-e-books.com/index.html

The American Cancer Society – A list of Herbs, Vitamins and Minerals under the Complementary and Alternative Medicine category.
www.cancer.org/treatment/treatmentsandsideeffects/complementaryandalternativemedicine/herbsvitaminsandminerals/index

"The New Prostate Cancer Nutrition Book". Dr Charles "Snuffy" Myers. http://www.prostateforum.com/nutrition-book.html.

The US National Cancer Institute's comments on pomegranate juice.
www.cancer.gov/cancertopics/pdq/cam/prostatesupplements/healthprofessional/page5.

Chapter 15.   The Role of Support Groups
The "Informed Prostate Cancer Support Group" (IPCSG).
http://www.ipcsg.org/

Us Too International www.ustoo.org

Chapter 22.   How Do You Get to a Final Treatment Decision?
Dr John McHugh's Decision Worksheet/Cheat Sheet.
http://theprostatedecision.wordpress.com/mchugh-decision-worksheetcheatsheet/

Appendix 4.
Reference Listings
Chapter 1. I am Diagnosed with Prostate Cancer
1. Bratt O, et al., **Hereditary Prostate Cancer: Clinical Aspects.** The Journal of Urology, Vol. 168, 906–913, September 2002.

Chapter 2. What is Prostate Cancer?
1. Australian Institute of Health and Welfare. Incidence and Prevalence of Chronic Disease, 2009. http://www.aihw.gov.au/cdarf/data_pages/incidence_prevalence/index.cfm#Diabetes.

Chapter 3. How is Prostate Cancer Detected?
1. Thompson IM, et al., **Prevalence of prostate cancer among men with a PSA level < or =4.0 ng per millilitre.** New England Journal of Medicine, 2004; 350(22): 2239-46.
2. Boots WebMD Web site. **Prostate Cancer Guide.** www.webmd.boots.com/prostatecancer/guide/psa-test-prostate-cancer.
3. See 1 and 2 above.
4. El Camino Urology Medical Group web site. **ProstateCancer.** www.elcaminourology.com/PSAandProstateCancer.html.
5. Scosyrev, E, et al., **PSA screening for prostate cancer and the risk of overt metastatic disease at presentation: Analysis of trends over time.** Cancer. 2012 Dec 1;118 (23):5768-76.
6. **Hunter Prostate Cancer Alliance web site.** www.hpca.org.au/pcfmenu/testingmenu/item/51-morepsa.html#Density
7. Prostate Health Index (*phi*). **FDA Approves New Blood Test to Improve Prostate Cancer Detection, June 2012.**
8. **Clinical Information about the 4Kscore Test.** OPKO Diagnostics. http://clinical.opko.com/how-does-4kscore-test-work.

9. **Pre-treatment Genetic Test Predicts Recurrence in Prostate Cancer.** http://www.onclive.com/web-exclusives/Pretreatment-Genetic-Test-Predicts-Recurrence-in-Prostate-Cancer#sthash.jlElkaKK.dpuf.
10. Castro E, Goh C, Saunders E, et al., **Germline BRCA Mutations Are Associated With Higher Risk of Nodal Involvement, Distant Metastasis, and Poor Survival Outcomes in Prostate Cancer.** JCO May 10, 2013 vol. 31 no. 14 1748-1757.
11. Pokorny MR, de Rooij M, et al., **Prospective Study of Diagnostic Accuracy Comparing Prostate Cancer Detection by Transrectal Ultrasound–Guided Biopsy Versus Magnetic Resonance (MR) Imaging with Subsequent MR-guided Biopsy in Men Without Previous Prostate Biopsies.** Eur Urol. 2014 Jul; 66(1):22-9.
12. Bonekamp D, Jacobs MA, El-Khouli R, et al., **Advancements in MR imaging of the prostate: from diagnosis to interventions.** Radiographics 31 (3 Suppl): 677–703. http://www.ncbi.nlm.nih.gov/pmc/articles/PMC3093638/.
13. Rothwax JT, George AK, et al., **Multiparametric MRI in Biopsy Guidance for Prostate Cancer: Fusion-Guided.** BioMed Research International, Volume 2014, Article ID 439171.
14. Bloch BN, Genega EM, Costa DN, et al., **Prediction of prostate cancer extracapsular extension with high spatial resolution dynamic contrast-enhanced 3-T MRI.** Eur Radiol. 2012 Oct; 22(10): 2201-10.
15. Barentsz JO, Richenberg J, Clements R, et al., **ESUR prostate MR guidelines 2012.** European Radiology 2012 10.1007/s00330-011-2377-y.
16. Junker D, Schäfer G, Edlinger M, et al., **Evaluation of the PI-RADS Scoring System for Classifying mpMRI Findings in Men with Suspicion of Prostate Cancer.** BioMed Research Int. Vol. 2013 (2013), Article ID 252939.

Chapter 4. Introductory Comments on Treatment Options
1. Jani AB, Hellman S. **Early prostate cancer: clinical decision-making.** Lancet 2003 Vol.: 361: 1243-52.

Chapter 5. Active Surveillance

1. Ip S, Dahabreh IJ, Chung M, et al., **An evidence review of active surveillance in men with localized prostate cancer.** Evid Rep Technol Assess (Full Rep). 2011 Dec; (204):1-341.
2. Mohler JL. Roswell Park Cancer Institute and chair of the NCCN Guidelines Panel for Prostate Cancer, **Presentation at the NCCN 16th Annual Conference in the USA.**
3. Klotz L, Zhang L, Lam A., et al. **Clinical results of long-term follow-up of a large active surveillance cohort with localised prostate cancer.** J Clin Oncol 2010; 28: 126–31.
4. Sung Kyu Hong. **Clinically insignificant prostate cancers: are they really insignificant?** http://approstate.org/workshop/201101/program/files/APPS_Sung%20Kyu%20Hong.pdf.
5. Wolters T, Roobol MJ, van Leeuwen PJ, et al., **A critical analysis of the tumour volume threshold for clinically insignificant prostate cancer using a data set of a randomized screening trial.** J Urol. 2011 Jan; 185(1): 121-5.
6. Jeldres C, Suardi N, Walz J, et al., **Validation of the contemporary Epstein criteria for insignificant prostate cancer in European men.** Eur Urol. 2008 Dec; 54(6): 1306-13. Epub 2007 Dec 7.
7. Mottet N, Bastian PJ, Bellmunt J, et al., **Pocket Guidelines on Prostate Cancer Updated April 2014.** European Urology Association.
8. See 5 above.

Chapter 6. Surgery

1. Rozet F, et al., Dept of Urology, Institut Montsouris, Paris, France. **A Direct Comparison of Robotic Assisted Versus Pure Laparoscopic Prostatectomy: A Single Institution's Experience.**
   http://www.abmedica.it/Rozet%20J%20Urol%202007.pdf
2. Lepor H. **Smilow Comprehensive Prostate Cancer Centre Web Site**
   http://prostatecancer.med.nyu.edu/treatment/prostate-cancer-surgery.

3. Walsh PC, Lepor H, Eggleston JC. **Radical prostatectomy with preservation of sexual function: anatomical and pathological considerations.** Prostate. 1983; 4(5): 473-85.
4. Marien T, Sankin A, Lepor H. **Factors predicting preservation of erectile function in men undergoing open radical retropubic prostatectomy.** J Urol. 2009 Apr; 181(4): 1817-22.
5. Jacobs EFP, Boris R, et al., **Advances in Robotic-Assisted Radical Prostatectomy over Time.** Prostate Cancer, Vol. 2013 (2013), Article ID 902686.
6. Ahlering T. Department of Urology, University of California, Irvine. http://www.urology.uci.edu/prostate/index.html.
7. Australian Institute of Health and Welfare. **Incidence and Prevalence of Chronic Disease, 2009.** www.aihw.gov.au/cdarf/data_pages/incidence_prevalence/index.cfm#Diabetes.
8. Park JJ, Kim CK, Park SY, et al., **Prostate Cancer: Role of Pre-treatment Multiparametric 3-T MRI in Predicting Biochemical Recurrence After Radical Prostatectomy.** AJR Am J Roentgenol. 2014; 202:W459-W465.

Chapter 7. Radiation
1. Frank SJ, Pisters LL, Davis J, et al., **An assessment of quality of life following radical prostatectomy, high dose external beam radiation therapy and brachytherapy iodine implantation as monotherapies for localized prostate cancer.** J Urol. 2007 Jun; 177(6): 2151-6; discussion 2156.
2. Prostate Cancer Foundation of Australia. **External Beam Radiotherapy.** http://www.prostate.org.au/articleLive/pages/External-BeamRadiotherapy.html.
3. Feng FY, Blas K, Olson K, et al., **Retrospective evaluation reveals that long-term androgen deprivation therapy improves cause-specific and overall survival in the setting of dose-escalated radiation for high-risk prostate cancer.** Int J Radiat Oncol Biol Phys. 2013 May 1; 86(1): 64-71.

4. **Erectile Dysfunction Guidance** web site: EBRT and Viagra.http://edguidance.com/viagra/.
5. Kosuri S, Aktar NH, Smith M, et al., **Review of Salvage Therapy for Biochemically Recurrent Prostate Cancer: The Role of Imaging and Rationale for Systemic Salvage Targeted Anti-Prostate-Specific Membrane Antigen Radioimmunotherapy.** Advances in Urology, Vol. 2012 (2012), Art ID 921674.
6. Pound CR, Partin AW, Eisenberger MA, et al., **Natural History of Progression after PSA Elevation Following Radical Prostatectomy.** JAMA 1999; 281:1591–7. PMID: 10235151.
7. Roehl KA, Han M, Ramos CG, et al., **Cancer Progression and Survival Rates Following Anatomical Radical Retropubic Prostatectomy in 3,478 Consecutive Patients: Long-Term Results.** *J Urol.* 2004; 172:910–14. PMID: 15310996.
8. See 5 above.
9. Garnick MB. **How to handle a relapse after treatment for prostate cancer.** Prostate Knowledge, Harvard Medical School. http://www.harvardprostateknowledge.org/ how-to-handle-a-relapse-after-treatment-for-prostate-cancer.
10. Mangar SA, Huddart RA, Parker CC, et al., **Technological advances in radiotherapy for the treatment of localised prostate cancer.** Eur J Cancer. 2005 Apr; 41(6): 908-21.
11. **IMRT for prostate cancer.** Cancer Centers of America web site. http://www.cancercenter.com/prostate-cancer/imrt/.
12. Kirichenko, A, et al., **IMRT versus 3D CRT for prostate cancer, new long-term data assesses side effects.** http://psychcentral.com/news/archives/2006-11/fccc-iv3110106.html.
13. Sharma, NK, Li, T., Chen, DY., et al., **IMRT Reduces Gastrointestinal Toxicity in Patients treated with ADT for Prostate Cancer.** *Int J Rad Onco•Biology•Physics 2011; 80 (2): 437-444.*

14. Zhou GX, Xu SP, Dai XK, et al., **Clinical dosimetric study of three radiotherapy techniques for postoperative breast cancer: Helical Tomotherapy, IMRT, and 3D-CRT.** Technol Cancer Res Treat. 2011 Feb; 10(1):15-23.
15. **RapidArc® - the next dimension in speed and precision.** http://www.varian.com/euen/oncology/treatments/treatment_techniques/rapidarc/.
16. **Stereotactic Body Radiotherapy for Primary Management of Early-Stage, Low- to Intermediate-Risk Prostate Cancer: Report of the American Society for Therapeutic Radiology and Oncology Emerging Technology Committee.** www.redjournal.org/article/S0360-3016(09)03543-3/fulltext
17. UCLA Health. Radiation Oncology UCLA. **Stereotactic Body Radiotherapy for Prostate Cancer.** http://radonc.ucla.edu/body.cfm?id=244.
18. King CR, James D. Brooks JD, et al., **Long-Term Outcomes from a Prospective Trial of Stereotactic Body Radiotherapy for Low-risk Prostate Cancer.** http://radonc.ucla.edu/workfiles/SBRT/Prostate_SBRT_Patient_Info.pdf
19. Yu JB, Cramer LD, Herrin J, et al., **SBRT Vs IMRT for Prostate Cancer: Comparison of Toxicity.** JCO March 10, 2014 JCO.2013.53.8652.
20. West Australian Dept. of Health. Sir Gairdner Hospital, Perth, West Australia, Australia. **CyberKnife Robotic Radiosurgery System Patient Information Sheet.** www.scgh.health.wa.gov.au/OurServices/CancerCentre/RadiationOncology/Patient/pdf/CyberKnifePatientInformationSheet.pdf.
21. Zietman AL, DeSilvio ML, Slater JD, et al., **Comparisons of conventional-dose vs high-dose conformal radiation therapy in clinically localized adenocarcinoma of the prostate: a randomized controlled trial.** J. A. M. A. 294 (10, 1233-1239 (2005).
22. Foote RL, Stafford SL, Petersen IA, et al., **The clinical case for proton beam therapy.** Radiation Oncology 2012, 7:174

23. Efstathiou JA. **A Landmark Study Compares Proton Beam Therapy with Standard Radiation Therapy.** Advances at Mass. General Cancer Center - Fall 2013. www.massgeneral.org/cancer/assets/advancesincancer/ADVQ413_Cancer_Proton%20Beam%20Therapy%20(2).pdf.
24. Talcott A, Rossi C, Shipley WU, et al., **Patient-Reported Long-term Outcomes After Conventional and High-Dose Combined Proton and Photon Radiation for Early Prostate Cancer.** JAMA. 2010; 303(11): 1046-1053.
25. As 21 above.
26. Chung CS, Keating N, Yock T, Tarbell N. **Comparative Analysis of Second Malignancy Risk in Patients Treated with Proton Therapy versus Conventional Photon Therapy.** Int J Radiat Oncol Biol Phys. Vol. 72, Supp, PS8, Sept 2008.
27. Fontenot JD, Lee AK, Newhauser WD. **Risk of secondary malignant neoplasms from proton therapy and intensity-modulated x-ray therapy for early-stage prostate cancer.** Int J Radiat Oncol Biol Phys. 2009 Jun 1; 74(2): 616-22.
28. Allen AM, Pawlicki T, Dong L. **An evidence based review of proton beam therapy: the report of ASTRO's emerging technology committee.** Radiother Oncol. 2012 Apr; 103(1): 8-11.
29. Efstathiou, JA, Gray PJ, Zietman AL. **Proton Beam Therapy and Localised Prostate Cancer: Current Status and Controversies.** British Journal of Cancer 108, no. 6 (April 2, 2013): 1225–1230.
30. Lawenda BD. Proton Beam Therapy: **The Rolls Royce of Radiation Oncology.** www.integrativeoncology-essentials.com/2013/03/proton-beam-therapy-the-rolls-royce-of-radiation-oncology/#sthash.6sONAuAD.aq4qTINH.dpuf.
31. Grimm P, Billiet I, Bostwick D, et al., **Comparative analysis of prostate-specific antigen free survival outcomes for patients with low, intermediate and high risk prostate cancer treatment by radical therapy. Results from the Prostate Cancer Results Study Group.** BJU Int. 2012 Feb; 109 Suppl 1:22-9.

32. Langley SEM, Laing RW. **4D Brachytherapy - a novel real-time prostate brachytherapy technique using stranded and loose seeds.** BJU Int. Vol. 109, Issue Supp s1, pages 1–6, Feb 2012. http://www.4dbrachytherapy.com/index.php/overview.
33. Hsu I-Chow, Yamada Y, Vigneault E, Pouliot J. **Generalized Criteria for the use of Brachytherapy in the treatment of Prostate Cancer August 2008.** American Brachytherapy Society Prostate High-Dose Rate Task Group. www.americanbrachytherapy.org/guidelines/HDRTaskGroup.pdf.

Chapter 8. Hyperthermia

1. Lieberman S. **A Review of Whole Body Hyperthermia and the Experience of Klinik St.Georg,** Townsend Letter, Aug/Sept 2009, http://kstg.net/e/publications/pdf/a_review_of_whole_body_hyperthermia_and_the_experience_of_klinik-st-georg.html.
2. van der Zee J., **Heating the patient: a promising approach?** Ann Oncol. 2002 Aug; 13(8):1173-84.
3. Douwes FR, Lieberman S., **Radiofrequency Transurethral Hyperthermia and Complete Androgen Blockade.** Jnl of Alternative & Complementary Therapies 7:6: 291-295, 2001.
4. Oleson RO, Samulski TV, Leopold KA, et al., **Sensitivity of hyperthermia trial outcomes to temperature and time: Implications for thermal goals of treatment.** Int Jour of Rad Onco*Biol*Physics Vol. 25, Issue 2, 15 Jan 1993.
5. **The Science of Hyperthermia,** Albathermia Web Site, www.albahyperthermia.com/hyperthermia-overview.html.
6. Falk MH, Issels RD., **Hyperthermia in oncology.** Int J Hyperthermia. 2001 Jan-Feb; 17(1):1-18.

Chapter 9. Cryosurgery

1. Babaian RJ, Donnelly B, Bahn D, et al. (Panel Members). **Best Practice Policy Statement on Cryosurgery for the Treatment of Localized Prostate Cancer.** American Urological Association.
www.auanet.org/education/guidelines/cryosurgery.cfm.
2. Heidenreich A, **Locally Recurrent Prostate Cancer Following Radiation Therapy: To Cut orTo Freeze?** European Urology, Volume 64 Issue 1, July 2013, Pages 8-10.
3. Bahn DK, Lee F, Badalament R, et al., **Targeted Cryoablation of the Prostate: 7-Year Outcomes in the Primary Treatment of Prostate Cancer.** Urology Vol 60, (Suppl 2A): 3–11, 2002.
4. Prof. John Kearsley, Director of the Prostate Cancer Institute,St George Hospital, Sydney, Australia. **Comments on the Institute's web site.**
http://www.prostatecancer.org.au/PCI/News.html.
5. Onik G, Vaughan D, Lotenfoe R, et al., **"Male lumpectomy": focal therapy for prostate cancer using cryoablation.** Urology. 2007 Dec; 70(6 Suppl): 16-21.

Chapter 10. High Intensity Focussed Ultrasound

1. Roundy N. **HIFU Treatment Data is Maturing.** PCRI Insights, March 2011, Vol. 14: No 1. http://prostate-cancer.org/PDFs/Is14-1_p14-20.pdf.
2. Brosman S. **HIFU – Not Ready For Prime Time.** PCRI Insights, March 2011, Vol. 14: No 1.
3. Lukka H, Waldron T, Chin J, et al., **High-intensity focused ultrasound for prostate cancer: a systematic review.** Clin Oncol (R Coll Radiol). 2011 Mar; 23(2): 117-27.
4. Ahmed HU, Freeman A, Kirkham A. **Focal therapy for localized prostate cancer: a phase I/II trial.** J Urol. 2011 Apr; 185(4): 1246-54.
5. Hindley RG, Dickinson L, Freeman A. **Focal therapy for localised unifocal and multifocal prostate cancer: a prospective development study.** The Lancet Oncology, Vol. 13, Issue 6, Pg 622 - 632, June 2012.

6. Cordeiro ER, Cathelineau X, Thüroff S, et al., **High-intensity focused ultrasound (HIFU) for definitive treatment of prostate cancer.** BJU Int. 2012 Nov; 110(9): 1228-42.
7. Obyn C, Mambourg F. **Assessment of high intensity focused ultrasound for the treatment of prostate cancer.** Acta Chir Belg. 2009 Oct; 109(5): 581-6.
8. Dickinson L, Hu Y, Ahmed HU, et al. **Image-Directed, Tissue Preserving Focal Therapy of Prostate Cancer: a Feasibility Study of a Novel Deformable MR-US Registration System.** BJU Int. Vol. 112, Issue 5, pages 594–601, Sept 2013.
9. Scionti S. **Targeted Focal Prostate Cancer Treatment.** Scionti Prostate Centre Web Site: www.drscionti.com/targeted-focal-prostate-cancer-treatment.

Chapter 11. Focal Laser Ablation
1. **Smilow Comprehensive Prostate Cancer Center,** NYULMC: http://prostate-cancer.med.nyu.edu/treatment/focal-laser-ablation-prostate-cancer.
2. Turkbey B, Ravizzini G, Mani H, et al.,**3T MR Imaging of the Prostate Gland: What the Urologist Needs to Know.** National Cancer Institute, NIH, USA. www.baristurkbey.com/images/prostate%20poster.pdf.
3. Costa DN, Bloch BN, Yao DF, et al.,**Diagnosis of relevant prostate cancer using supplementary cores from magnetic resonance imaging-prompted areas following multiple failed biopsies.** Magnetic Resonance Imaging Jul 2013, 31(6); 947-952.
4. Sperling D, **Sperling Prostate Centre** http://sperlingprostatecenter.com/
5. Oto A, Sethi I, Karczmar G, et al., **MR imaging-guided focal laser ablation for prostate cancer: phase I trial.** Radiology. 2013 Jun; 267(3): 932-40.
6. **Smilow Comprehensive Prostate Cancer Center,** NYULMC: http://prostate-cancer.med.nyu.edu/treatment/focal-laser-ablation-prostate-cancer.

7. Mottet N, Bastian PJ, Bellmunt J, et al., **Guidelines on Prostate Cancer Updated April 2014.** European UrologyAssociation. http://www.uroweb.org/gls/pdf/1607%20Prostate%20Cancer_LRV3.pdf.
8. Mottet N, Bastian PJ, Bellmunt J, et al., **Pocket Guidelines on Prostate Cancer Updated April 2014.** European Urology Association. http://www.uroweb.org/gls/pockets/english/PCProstate%20Cancer_LR.pdf

Chapter 12. Hormone Therapy

1. **Xtandi Phase 111 Clinical Trial Web Site.** https://www.xtandihcp.com/phase-3-trial-design.
2. Kantoff PW, Higano CS, Shore ND, et al., **Sipuleucel-T Immunotherapy for Castration-Resistant Prostate Cancer.** New England Journal of Medicine. Vol. 363 No. 5; July 2010.
3. **Abiraterone: a story of scientific innovation and commercial partnership.** Institute of Cancer Research, UK. http://www.icr.ac.uk/press/recent_featured_articles/Story_Abiraterone/index.shtml.
4. Perlmutter MA, Lepor H. **Androgen Deprivation Therapy in the Treatment of Advanced Prostate Cancer.** Rev Urol 2007; 9(Suppl 1): S3-S8.
5. See 4 above.

Chapter 13. Chemotherapy and Immunotherapy

1. **Metastatic Cancer.** National Cancer Institute Fact Sheet. http://www.cancer.gov/cancertopics/factsheet/Sites-Types/metastatic.
2. **What biophosphonates are.** Cancer Research UK. http://www.cancerresearchuk.org/cancer-help/about-cancer/treatment/bisphosphonate/what-bisphosphonates-are.

3. Sartor O, Eisenberger M, Kattan MW, et al., **Unmet Needs in the Prediction and Detection of Metastates in Prostate Cancer.** The Oncologist Express, May 6, 2013.
4. Sweeney C, Chen Y, Carducci MA, et al., **Impact on overall survival (OS) with chemo-hormonaltherapy versus hormonal therapy for hormone-sensitive newly metastatic prostate cancer (mPrCa): an ECOG-led phase III randomized trial.** J Clin Oncol. 2014; 32:5s (suppl; abstr LBA2).
5. **Bavarian Nordic Initiates Pivotal Phase 3 Trial of PROSTVAC® Prostate Cancer Immunotherapy.** http://ci.bavarian-nordic.com/media/news.aspx?news=1919.
6. Simpson RJ, Lim JW, Moritz RL, Mathivanan S. **Exosomes: proteomic insights and diagnostic potential.** Expert Rev Proteomics. 2009 Jun; 6(3): 267-83.
7. Giusti I, Dolo V. **Extracellular vesicles in prostate cancer: new future clinical strategies?** Biomed Res Int. 2014; 2014: 561571.

Chapter 14. Complementary and Alternative Therapies

1. Lee MS, Ernst E. **Systematic reviews of t'ai chi: an overview.** Br J Sports Med. Aug 2012 46(10): 713-8.
2. Madsen MV, Gøtzsche PC, Hróbjartsson A. **Acupuncture treatment for pain: systematic review of randomised clinical trials with acupuncture, placebo acupuncture, and no acupuncture groups.** BMJ. 2009 Jan 27; 338:a3115.
3. Macdonald R, Tacklind JW, Rutks I, Wilt TJ. **Serenoa repens monotherapy for benign prostatic hyperplasia (BPH): an updated Cochrane systematic review.** BJU Int. Vol. 109, Issue 12, pages 1756–1761, June 2012.
4. Khana N, Adhamia VM, Mukhtara HV. **Review: Green Tea Polyphenols in Chemoprevention of Prostate Cancer: Preclinical and Clinical Studies.** Nutrition and Cancer, Volume 61, Issue 6, 2009.

5. Liua J, Yu H, Jin F, Kondoa R, Zhang C, et al., **Stereospecificity of hydroxyl group at C-20 in antiproliferative action of ginsenoside Rh2 on prostate cancer cells.** Fitoterapia, Volume 81, Issue 7, October 2010.
6. Wang W, Rayburn ER, Hao M, et al., **Experimental therapy of prostate cancer with novel natural product anti-cancer ginsenosides.** Prostate. 2008 Jun 1; 68(8): 809-19.
7. Wang W, Wang H, Rayburn ER, et al., **20(S)-25-methoxyl-dammarane-3beta, 12beta, 20-triol, a novel natural product for prostate cancer therapy: activity in vitro and in vivo and mechanisms of action.** Br J Cancer. 2008 Feb 26; 98(4): 792-802.
8. von Holtz RL, Fink CS, Awad AB. **beta-Sitosterol activates the sphingomyelin cycle and induces apoptosis in LNCaP human prostate cancer cells.** Nutr Cancer. 1998; 32(1): 8-12.
9. Awad AB, Burr AT, Fink CS.**Effect of resveratrol and beta-sitosterol in combination on reactive oxygen species and prostaglandin release by PC-3 cells.** Prostaglandins Leukot Essent Fatty Acids 72 (3): 219-26, 2005.
10. Obermüller-Jevic UC, Olano-Martin E, Corbacho AM, et al., **Lycopene inhibits the growth of normal human prostate epithelial cells in vitro.** J Nutr. 2003 Nov; 133(11): 3356-60.
11. Medina MA. **Glutamine and Cancer.** J. Nutr. September 1, 2001 vol. 131 no. 9 2539S-2542S.
12. Zhang X-K. **Vitamin A and apoptosis in prostate cancer.** Endocrine-Related Cancer (2002) 9 87–102.
13. Gaziano JM, Sesso HD, Christen WG, et al., **Multivitamins in the prevention of cancer in men: the Physicians' Health Study II randomized controlled trial.** JAMA. 2012 Nov 14; 308(18): 1871-80.
14. Ho E. **Zinc and Antioxidants in Cancer Chemoprevention.** Linus Pauling Institute, Oregon State University. http://lpi.oregonstate.edu/CCP/zinc-cancer.html.

15. Richman EL, Kenfield SA, Chavarro JE, et al., **Men With Prostate Cancer Should Eat Healthy Vegetable Fats.** UC San Francisco. JAMA Internal Medicine on line 10 June 2013.
16. Richman EL, Kenfield SA, Chavarro JE, et al., **Fat Intake After Diagnosis and Risk of Lethal Prostate Cancer and All-Cause Mortality.** JAMA Intern Med. 2013; 173(14): 1318-1326.
17. Stacewicz-Sapuntzakis M, Borthakur G, Burns JL, Bowen PE. **Correlations of dietary patterns with prostate health.** Mol Nutr Food Res. 2008 Jan; 52(1): 114-30.
18. Itsiopoulos C, Hodge A, Kaimakamis, M. **Can the Mediterranean diet prevent prostate cancer?** Mol Nutr Food Res. 2009 Feb; 53(2):227-39.
19. Sonoda T, Nagata Y, Mori M, et al., **A case-control study of diet and prostate cancer in Japan: possible protective effect of traditional Japanese diet.** Cancer Sci. 2004 Mar; 95(3): 238-42.
20. Mori M, Masumori N, Fukuta F, et al., **Traditional Japanese diet and prostate cancer.** Mol Nutr Food Res. 2009 Feb; 53(2):191-200.
21. Pantuck AJ, Leppert JT, Zomorodian N, et al., **Phase II Study of Pomegranate Juice for Men with Rising PSA following Surgery or Radiation for Prostate Cancer.** Clinical Cancer Research (Vol. 12 p 4018-4026) 2006.
22. Jonas WB, Gaddipati JP, Rajeshkumar NV, et al., **Can homeopathic treatment slow prostate cancer growth?** Integr Cancer Ther. 2006 Dec; 5(4):343-9.
23. **Shark Cartilage.** American Cancer Society. www.cancer.org/treatment/treatmentsandsideeffects/complementaryandalternativemedicine/pharmacologicalandbiologicaltreatment/shark-cartilage.
24. Adlerova L, Bartoskova A, Faldyna M. **Lactoferrin: a review.** Veterinarni Medicina, 53, 2008(9): 457–468.
25. Gibbons JA, Kanwar RK, Kanwar JR. **Lactoferrin and cancer in different cancer models.** Front Biosci (Schol Ed). 2011 Jun 1; 3:1080-8.

Chapter 15. The Role of Support Groups
1. Marckini R. *Brotherhood of the Balloon*. www.protonbob.com/proton-treatment-homepage.asp.

Chapter 21. Enter the Case for Hyperthermia
1. Douwes FR, Lieberman S., Radiofrequency Transurethral Hyperthermia and Complete Androgen Blockade. Jnl of Alternative & Complementary Therapies 7:6: 291-295, 2001.

Appendix 5.

Proton Beam Centres

Proton Beam Therapy is regarded by sections of the medical fraternity as being an experimental technique with outcomes not fully confirmed by long term randomized controlled studies. PBT is the most advanced radiation therapy technique available today and continues to rapidly progress from a technological standpoint. The relatively small number of centres world-wide, also contribute to general ignorance of the technique amongst general practitioners and even urologists and radiation oncologists in almost every country. This star wars-like technology has been used in the treatment of malignant and benign tumours since the 1950's. As of 2011, over 73,000 patients have been treated at proton beam treatment centres around the world. By mid-2015 this number will have grown to more than 100,000 patients. The number of these centres is growing quickly with around 31 presently treating patients for prostate cancer and another 10 likely to start treating patients during 2014 and 2015.

There are a small number of Proton Beam Centres around the world that are fixed beam systems that only treat cancers of the eye or the head or neck. These facilities are omitted from the following listings.

Presently Treating Prostate Cancer Patients

James M. Slater, M.D. Proton Treatment and Research Centre, Loma Linda University Medical Centre, California

http://www.protons.com/proton-therapy/why-choose-lomalinda/our-center.pagetre

Address: 11155 Mountain View Avenue, Loma Linda, California 92354, USA.

Phone: +1-800-776-8667 or +1 (909) 558 3422

The first and most experienced Proton Beam Centre in the world. They have treated more than 17,500 patients since they opened 24 years ago. In 1990 James M. Slater, MD, pioneered the field of proton therapy at Loma Linda University Medical Centre (LLUMC) and it remained the only hospital-based treatment centre of its kind in the United States until 2003. It has treated 12,000 prostate cancer patients in the 24 years. It is interesting to note that 51% of all patients (all cancer forms) were older than 65 years; 34% were in the age group 55 to 64; 9% were 45 to 54 and 6% were younger than 45 years old.

It clinical proton therapy team has the following combined years of experience:

Physicians 170+ years; Physicists and Dosimetrists 270+ years and Therapists 350+ years.

The LLUMC has conducted more clinical trials on more tumour sites and published more long term clinical outcomes than any other proton beam centre in the world.

The University of Florida Proton Therapy Institute. Florida

http://www.floridaproton.org/

Address: 2015 North Jefferson Street, Jacksonville, Florida 32206, USA

Phone: +1 (904) 588 1800

Since opening in August 2006, more than 150,000 proton cancer treatments have been delivered to more than 4,377 patients at the University of Florida Proton Therapy Institute, ranking the facility among the top 10 proton therapy centres worldwide for the number of patients treated.

M.D. Anderson Cancer Centre's Proton Centre, Houston

http://www.mdanderson.org/patient-and-cancer-information/proton-therapy-center/index.html

Address: The University of Texas MD Anderson Cancer Centre, 1515 Holcombe Blvd, Houston, Texas 77030, USA.

Phone: +1 (713) 792 2121 or ask MDAnderson: +1 (877) 632 6789

Since treating their first patient in May 2006, the dedicated team at the Proton Therapy Centre has helped countless patients overcome cancer and get back to living their lives. Since then they have treated nearly 2,100 men for prostate cancer with proton therapy.

The M.D. Anderson Cancer Centre's Proton Therapy Centre pioneered pencil beam scanning proton therapy treatment and currently (May 2014) is the only centre in the United States and one of only three clinical centres in the world using this technology to treat patients.

ProCure Proton Therapy Centre, Oklahoma City

www.procure.com/ContactUs/ContactUsOklahomaCity.aspx

Address: 5901 W. Memorial Road, Oklahoma City, Oklahoma 73142 USA.

Phone: +1 (888) 847 2640; from outside the USA: +1 (405) 773 6767

The ProCure Proton Therapy Centre in Oklahoma is one of three such centres operated by ProCure. The Oklahoma facility opened in July 2009 and by September 2011 had treated its 500th patient.

The Roberts Proton Therapy Centre, University of PA Health System, Philadelphia

http://www.pennmedicine.org/radiation-oncology/patient-care/treatments/proton-therapy/roberts-proton-therapy-center.html

Address: Perelman Centre for Advanced Medicine, 3400 Civic Centre Boulevard, Philadelphia, Pennsylvania 19104, USA.

Phone: +1 800-789-7366

The Roberts Proton Therapy Centre on its web site claims to be the largest such facility in the world with 4 gantry systems and a fixed-beam treatment room. It is housed within Penn Radiation Oncology and is seamlessly integrated with a full range of cancer services provided by Penn's Abramson Cancer Centre. It is a 75,000 square foot facility within the Perelman Centre for Advanced Medicine.

Hampton University Proton Therapy Institute, Virginia

http://www.hamptonproton.org/

Address: 40 Enterprise Pkwy, Hampton, Virginia 23666, USA.

Phone: +1 (757) 251 6800

The Hampton University Proton Therapy Institute (HUMPTI) opened in 2010 and its 5 treatment rooms were completed in 2011. It claims to be the world's largest free-standing proton beam facility. It treats about 1500 patients per year for a wide range of cancers. In early 2013 it formed a strategic alliance with Strategic Alliance Holdings, LLC (SAH) to treat cancer patients from the Middle East and North Africa which includes 32 countries.

CDH Proton Centre, Chicago Area, Illinois

http://www.cdhprotoncenter.com/

Address: 4455 Weaver Parkway, Warrenville, Illinois 60555, USA.

Phone: +1 (877) 887 5807

It is one of the three ProCure Proton Beam Therapy centres in the United States. The CDH Proton Centre is the first and only proton radiation centre in Illinois using state-of-the-art technology to treat adults and children with tumours and cancer from all over the world.

IU Health Proton Therapy Centre, Bloomington, Indiana

http://iuhealth.org/newsroom/listing/category/proton-therapy/

Address: 2425 N. Milo B. Sampson Lane, Bloomington, Indiana 47408, USA.

Phone: +1 (866) 487 6774

The IU Health Proton Therapy Centre celebrated its 10th anniversary of the treatment of its first patient, in February 2014. Originally incorporated as the Midwest Proton Radiotherapy Institute, or MPRI, by the IU Advanced Research and Technology Institute, or ARTI (now the IU Research and Technology Corporation, or IURTC), it was at the time one of only three proton centres in the USA.

Some 36% of the almost 2000 patients treated at the facility to date have been treated for prostate cancer. The facility treats patients from all around the world, but 86% of those undergoing therapy are from the US Midwest region.

Francis H. Burr Proton Centre, Boston

http://www.massgeneral.org/radiationoncology/BurrProtonCenter.aspx

Address: Francis H. Burr Proton Therapy Centre, 30 Fruit Street, Boston, Massachusetts 02114, USA.

Phone: +1 (617) 724 1680

The facility has two treatment rooms and is part of the Massachusetts General Hospital.

New Jersey/Metro New York ProCure Proton Therapy Centre, New Jersey

http://www.procure.com/ContactUs/ContactUsNewJersey.aspx

Address: 103 Cedar Grove Lane, Somerset, New Jersey 08873, USA.

Phone: +1 (877) 967 7628

ProCure has joined with CentraState Healthcare System and Princeton Radiation Oncology to ensure patients have a seamless and integrated experience. It is one of the three ProCure Proton Beam Centres in the USA.

ProCure SCCA Proton Therapy Centre, Seattle, Washington

http://www.procure.com/OurLocations/Seattle/ExploretheCenter.asp
Address: 1570 North 115th Street, Seattle, Washington 98133, USA.

Phone: +1 (877) 897 7628 (US Patients); +1 (206) 306 2800 (International Patients)

It is a partnership between ProCure and the SCCA Proton Therapy Seattle Cancer Care Alliance, Seattle, WA and is located on UW Medicine's Northwest Hospital & Medical Centre campus. The facility has three treatment rooms (one a fixed beam room; one a fixed beam room with the beam orientated at 60 degrees and a gantry room that provides 360 degree rotation).

The Provision Proton Therapy Centre, Knoxville, Tennessee

http://www.provisionproton.com/

Address: 6450 Provision Cares Way, Knoxville, Tennessee 37909, USA.

Phone: +1 (865) 862 1600

The Provision Centre for Proton Therapy is a member of Provision Health Alliance, nestled in the beautiful Dowell Springs campus in the heart of Knoxville. Its 90,000 square foot facility has the capability to treat up to 1,500 patients each year, and includes three treatment rooms with the latest proton therapy treatment equipment. The centre also houses two additional treatment rooms for the research and development of the ProNova SC360, a lower-cost, smaller, lighter and more energy efficient proton therapy solution that will soon come to market, making proton therapy more affordable and accessible to treat a greater population of cancer patients.

Phone: +1 (212) 599 5555

Barnes Jewish Hospital, St. Louis, Missouri

http://www.siteman.wustl.edu

Address: 224 South Euclid Avenue, St. Louis, Missouri

Phone: +1 (314) 286 1222

The S. Lee Kling Proton Therapy Centre treated their first patient in December 2013. It is the first centre in the world to install the Mevion S250 Proton Therapy System from Mevion Medical Systems, Inc. of Littleton, Massachusetts. This installation is the first of a new generation of Proton Therapy systems with similar treatment options to earlier systems, but with a greatly reduced physical footprint, streamline clinical workflows and greatly reduced implementation and operating costs.

The Scripps Proton Therapy Centre, San Diego, California

http://www.scripps.org/services/cancer-care__proton-therapy

Address: 9730 Summers Ridge Road, San Diego, California 92121, USA.

Phone: +1 (858) 549 7400

Scripps Proton Therapy Centre offers five treatment rooms, all of which feature pencil-beam scanning technology. Pencil-beam scanning allows the clinical team to manipulate the protons so their energy conforms to each tumour's unique shape. Three of the five treatment room include 360 degree gantries which allow the selection of an optimum angle of proton radiation to a tumour. The latest suite of imaging tools within the facility include MRI, PET – CT and 4D CT.

Willis-Knighton Proton Therapy Centre, Shreveport, Louisiana

http://www.wkhs.com/Cancer/Cancer-Treatment-Services/Proton-Therapy

Address: 2600 Kings Highway, Shreveport, Louisiana 71103, USA.

Phone: +1 (318) 212 8300

The Centre treated its first patients in September 2014. The Centre is the first in the world to use the Proteous One intensity modulated pencil beam technology, which is considered by the staff at the Willis-Knighton Proton Therapy Centre to be game changing.

USA – Under Construction - Opening in 2014 or early 2015

The McLaren Proton Therapy Centre, Flint, Michigan (under construction – Radiance 330 Proton Therapy System)

http://www.mclaren.org/protontherapy/protontherapy.aspx

Address: G-4100 Beecher Road, Flint, Michigan 48532, USA.

Phone: +1 (855) 697 7686 or +1 (810) 342 3840

The McLaren Proton Therapy Centre is a partnership between McLaren Health Care and ProTom International, Inc., a Texas-based healthcare technology company. The Centre represents the next generation of proton therapy centres with several advances in design and technology. The three gantry treatment rooms will share the proton beam, generated by the Radiance 330 Synchrotron manufactured by ProTom International. Each of the three gantries will have a pencil beam scanning nozzle and the latest in room CT and X-Ray scanning capabilities.

The shielding walls and lids surrounding the synchrotron, proton beam line and treatment area are one-half, to one-third the thickness of first-generation proton centres.

UF Health Cancer Centre at Orlando Health Proton Therapy Centre, Orlando, Florida (under construction – Mevion S250)

http://www.orlandohealth.com

Address: 1400 S. Orange Avenue, Orlando, Florida 32806, USA

Phone: +1 (321) 843 2584

The 15,000 square foot facility is scheduled to open in early 2015 It will accommodate the Mevion S250 superconducting synchrocyclotron proton accelerator. It expects to treat 30 patients a day.

Robert Wood Johnson University Hospital, New Jersey (under testing – Mevion S250)

http://www.rwjuh.edu/patient_guide/patients.html

Address: One Robert Wood Johnson Place, New Brunswick, New Jersey 08901, USA

Phone: +1 (732) 828 3000

The facility is due to start treating patients during 2014 after taking delivery of a Mevion S250 Proton Therapy System in July 2012.

First Coast Oncology, Jacksonville, Florida (under construction – Mevion S250 system already delivered)

http://www.firstcoastoncology.com/proton-therapy

Address: 10881 San Jose Boulevard, Jacksonville, Florida 32223, USA

Phone: +1 (904) 880 5522

This is the first privately physician-funded proton therapy system in the United States.

The Stephenson Cancer Centre, Oklahoma University, Oklahoma City, Oklahoma (under construction – Mevion S250)

http://www.oumedicine.com/cancer

Address: 800 NE 10th Street, Oklahoma City, Oklahoma 73104, USA

Phone: +1 (855) 750 2273

They are presently installing the first of two Mevion S250 Proton Therapy Systems, which is the first of a new generation of lower cost Proton Therapy Systems from Mevion Medical Systems, Inc.

USA - Under Construction – Opening Later than mid-2015

Mayo Clinic Proton Beam Therapy Program

http://www.mayoclinic.org/proton-beam-therapy

The Mayo Clinic presently has two proton beam therapy centres under construction in Rochester, Minnesota and Phoenix, Arizona. The first treatment rooms will be available for patients in Rochester in the summer of 2015 and in Arizona in 2016. All eight treatment rooms will be operational by 2017. They will incorporate the latest pencil beam scanning technology.

University Hospitals, Seidman Cancer Centre, Cleveland, Ohio (under construction – Mevion S250)

http://www.uhhospitals.org.seidman

Address: 11100 Euclid Avenue, Cleveland, Ohio 44106, USA

Phone: +1 (866) 844 2273

This facility will start treating patients in 2015.

Maryland Proton Treatment Centre, Baltimore, Maryland (under construction)

https://www.pennmedicine.org/s-

Address: 850 W. Baltimore Street, Baltimore, Maryland 21201, USA

Phone: +1 (410) 706 7590

This facility will be housed in an all-new 100000 square foot facility that will have five treatment rooms (four gantries and one fixed beam system). The centre expects to open in mid-2015.

Texas Proton Therapy Centre LLC, Dallas, Texas (under construction)

Opening in 2015 with an IBA system with two gantry rooms and one fixed-beam room.

The Emory Proton Therapy Centre, Winship Cancer Institute, Atlanta, Georgia (under construction)

https://winshipcancer.emory.edu/patient-care/clinics-and-centers/proton-therapy-center.html

Address: 1365 Clifton Road NE, Bldg. C, Atlanta, Georgia 30322, USA

Phone: +1 (404) 778-1900

To be opened in 2016. It will be equipped with 5 Varian ProBeam Technology treatment rooms.

USA - Planned Facilities

Todd Cancer Pavilion Long Beach Memorial Hospital, California

http://www.memorialcare.org/services/cancer-care/cancer-care-long-beach-memorial

Address: 2810 Long Beach Boulevard, Long Beach, California 90806, USA

Phone: +1 (562) 933 0900

This facility has contracted to install a Mevion S250 Proton Therapy System.

Dallas Proton Treatment Centre, The University of Texas Southwestern Medical Centre, Texas (awaiting ground breaking)

Tufts University School of Medicine, Boston, Massachusetts

UCSD Proton/Particle Treatment and Research Centre, San Diego, California (awaiting ground breaking)

Other Countries

China

Wanjie Proton Therapy Centre, Zibo, China

This facility started treating patients in late 2004. It has one gantry room plus a fixed beam room Their radiation oncologists and therapists were trained at the Massachusetts General Hospital in Boston, USA and their medical engineering staff were trained by IBA in Belgium.

Beijing Proton Medical Centre, Beijing, China

http://www.concordmedical.com/ourhospitals/bpmc.shtml

Address: 18/F, Tower A, Global Trade Centre, 36 North Third Ring Road East, Dongcheng District, Beijing, People's Republic of China, 100013

Phone: +86 10-5903-6688

The facility, built adjacent to the China-Japan Friendship Hospital in Beijing, Started treating patients in 2013.

Czech Republic

Proton Therapy Centre s.r.o., Prague, Czech Republic

http://www.proton-cancer-treatment.com

Address: Budinova 2437/1a, Prague 8, 180 00, Czech Republic

Phone: +42 (0) 222 999 000

This centre that has been in operation since December 2012 has 5 treatment rooms, including a fixed beam room and is supported by a full array of diagnostic equipment including CT, MRI and a PET/CT camera. The centre offers international patients full services and arranges accommodation and transport to and from the centre during the treatment period. Their proton therapy system utilises the latest pencil beam scanning techniques. They also maintain a UK web site to promote their services to British patients. See http://www.ukprotontherapy.co.uk

France

Centre Antoine-Lacassagne (CAL), Nice (under construction)

http://www.centreantoinelacassagne.org/fr

Address: 227 Avenue de la Lanterne, 06200 Nice, France

Phone: +33 (0) 4 92 03 10 80

Their proton therapy unit is under construction and will house an IBA Proteous One system.

Centre de Protontherapie de l'Instit Curie

http://protontherapie.curie.fr/

Address: Institut Curie, 26 rue d'ulm 75248, Paris cedex 05, France

Phone: +33 (0) 1 69 29 87 00

The facility opened in 2009. It recently upgraded the two fixed beam rooms with a new cyclotron and a gantry room.

Germany

West German Proton Therapy Centre Essen, WPE

http://www.uk-essen.de/wpe/english/home.html

Address: Hufelandstrasse 55, 45147 Essen, Germany

Phone: +49 (0)201 72255 – 209

The first of four treatment rooms for cancer therapy with protons at the WPE has already been commissioned. Gradually, the further three treatment rooms will follow.

Rinecker Proton Therapy Centre

http://www.rptc.de/

Address: Franz-von-Rinecker Strasse, 81371 Munich, Germany

Phone: +49 (0) 89 660 680

The Rinecker Therapy Centre is regarded as Europe's most prominent Proton Beam Therapy centre. Its facilities include four gantry systems as well as a fixed beam system. The latest imaging systems include

MRI, CT-PET and CT. The RPTC is the first large proton therapy centre in Europe to offer a complete hospital setting and comprehensive therapeutic options. Additionally, it is the first clinic in Germany that is also state-licensed for proton radiation treatment of patients with statutory health insurance.

University Hospital Carl Gustav Carus Dresden

http://www.uniklinikum-dresden.de/patienten-und-besucher/international-patients

Address: 01304 Dresden, Germany

Phone: +49 (0) 351 458 2036

The international department can assist with enquiries.

India

The Apollo Therapy Centre, Chennai (under construction)

http://www.apollohospitals.com/

Address: 21, Greams Lane, off Greams Road, Chennai – 600006, India

Phone: +91-44-28290200

It will start treating patients in 2016 and will include two gantry rooms and a fixed beam room. It will be equipped with pencil beam scanning technology.

Italy

ATrep – Agenziav Provinciale per la Protontherapia

http://www.atrep.provincia.tn.it

Address: via f.lli Perini 181, 38122 Trento TN), Italy

Phone: +46 (0) 1- 390409

The facility opened in 2013 and has an IBA two gantry room set up plus a fixed beam treatment room.

Japan

The National Cancer Centre, Kashiwa

http://www.ncc.go.jp/en/contact.html

Address: 6-5-1 Kashiwanoha, Kashiwa, Chiba 277-8577, Japan

Phone: +81 4 7133 1111

It has two gantry rooms and started treating patients in 1998. It was developed in association with Sumitomo Heavy Industry Ltd.

Shizuoka Cancer Centre, Shizuoka

http://www.scchr.jp/english/hospital/toha.html

Address: 1007 Shimonagakubo, Nagaizumi-cho, Sunto-gun, Shizuoka Prefecture 411-8777 Japan

Phone: +81-55-989-5222

Located against a backdrop of majestic Mount Fuji, the Shizuoka Cancer Center was opened in 2002 and offers top-class cancer treatment with cutting-edge medical technology and thorough support for patients.

Nagoya Proton Therapy Centre, Nagoya

http://www.nptc.city.nagoya.jp/english.html

Address: Nagoya City West Medical Centre, 1-1-1 Hirate-cho, Kita-ku, Nagoya, 462-8508, Japan

Phone: +81-52-991-8588

Uses the latest spot scanning techniques, provides an urban type environment for the patient and has the latest imaging technology all integrated to optimize treatment outcomes.

Medipolis Medical Research Institute

http://japanest-nippon.com/en/uniandins/us_detail.php?id=33

The Proton Beam Cancer Therapy Centre of the Medipolis Medical Research Institute started cancer treatment in 2011. It has a three gantry facility with one dedicated to breast cancer. The facility offers residential programs from US$36,000. The Proton Beam Cancer

Therapy Centre is highly regarded for its superior medical technologies, as well as for its dedicated efforts toward the eradication of cancer.

Southern Tohuko Proton Therapy Centre, Fukushima

http://www.southerntohoku-proton.com/english/greeting.html

Address: 172-7choume, Yatsuyamada, Koriyama, Fukushima 963-8563 JAPAN

This privately managed facility opened in 2008. Their prostate cancer protocol calls for delivery of a total radiation dosage of 74 -78 Grays over 37 to 39 treatments over 7.4 to 8 weeks.

Proton Medical Research Centre (PMRC), University of Tsukuba, Ibaraki

http://www.pmrc.tsukuba.ac.jp/engRadiotherapy.html

Address: 2-1-1 Amakubo, Tsukuba, Ibaraki 305-8576, Japan

Phone: +81-29-853-7100

Clinical treatments started with their two gantries in 2001. About 3,000 patients have been treated up until 2011, including about 300 treatments for prostate cancer.

Russia

Federal High-Technology Centre of Nuclear Medicine of FMBA, Dimitrovgrad

http://cluster-dgrad.ru

Address: 93, Khmelnitskogo Street, Dimitrovgrad, Ulyanovsk Region, Russia, 433508

Phone: 8 (84235) 4-82-45

It started treating patients via an IBA system with two gantry rooms and a fixed-beam room in 2013.

Sweden

Skandion Clinic, Uppsala (under construction)

http://www.skandionkliniken.se

The clinic is still under construction with first patients expected to be treated in 2015. The IBA system will have two gantry rooms and a fixed beam treatment room.

South Korea

The Proton Therapy Centre, National Cancer Centre, Ilsandong

http://www.nccproton.com/ or www.protonkorea.com (KMI International)

Address: 323 Ilsan-ro, Ilsandong – gu, Goyang – si, Gyeonggi – do, 410-769, Republic of Korea.

Phone: +82-31-920-1934

The Proton Therapy Centre opened in 2007 and has an IBA Porteous system that services three gantry rooms and a fixed-beam room. It treats Korean and international patients. KMI International work closely with the staff at the NCC to arrange first class treatment for international patients. This includes arranging top quality accommodation, daily transport, and a concierge service. (The author underwent prostate cancer treatment at the NCC in early 2013 at a cost of US$53,000 including accommodation).

Their senior professional staff were trained and worked in the United States and speak perfect English.

Switzerland

Paul Scherrer Institut, Villigen

http://p-therapie.web.psi.ch/e/index.html

Address: 5232 Villigen PSI, Switzerland

Phone: +41 56 310 21 11

PSI operates the first compact scanning-Gantry worldwide for proton radiation therapy of deep-seated tumours. The spot-scanning technique developed at PSI enables malignant tumours to be targeted with high precision deep inside in the body. They are at the leading edge of proton therapy research and are installing a second gantry to expand their treatment offering.

Taiwan

Chang Gung Memorial Hospital, Taipei

https://www.cgmh.org.tw/eng2002/about01.htm

Address: Administration Centre: No.199, Tunghwa Rd.,Taipei, Taiwan, Republic of China

Phone: + 88 6-2-27135211

Their Proton Beam facility started treating patients in 2012. No further details are available.

■■

Appendix 6.

Acknowledgements

I would like to thank my wife for giving me enormous support during my prostate cancer journey. Also, I thank her for her patience in my "absence in my study" for hundreds and hundreds of hours, whilst I researched and wrote this book. I am sure she became very tired of my singular focus on completing the "project".

My brother, Brian, gave me a generous insight into his treatment and as an accomplished author of over 45 eBooks published on his travels through many lands over three decades, gave me many valuable tips on getting this book published.

My two main proof readers, Felicity and Geoffrey did an excellent job. Felicity's focus was on English grammar, whilst Geoffrey focussed on the technology, particularly in the diagnostics and genetics areas.

My good friend John is thanked for introducing me to proton beam therapy and other prostate cancer sufferers that had different prostate cancer treatments, with differing outcomes.

I must thank the very busy members of the medical profession, who committed their valuable time to read the manuscript and to offer me suggestions for its improvement. It is appropriate to thank my doctors in Australia and at the NCC in Korea for their professional care and attention during my illness.

I thank my regular golfing partners, all of whom I badgered into reading the book to determine its 'readability'. Thanks also to 'Rob' for sharing his story with us in the last chapter of the book. He also gave interesting input after reading the book.

I hope that I have not overlooked anyone.

For more information go to www.anabcofprostatecancer.com.au.

Made in the USA
San Bernardino, CA
03 November 2015